CARDIOLOGY RESEARCH AND CLINICAL DEVELOPMENTS

CAROTID ARTERY DISEASE

RISK FACTORS, PROGNOSIS AND MANAGEMENT

CARDIOLOGY RESEARCH AND CLINICAL DEVELOPMENTS

Additional books in this series can be found on Nova's website under the Series tab.

Additional e-books in this series can be found on Nova's website under the e-book tab.

CAROTID ARTERY DISEASE

RISK FACTORS, PROGNOSIS AND MANAGEMENT

SHERRI DERRICKS
EDITOR

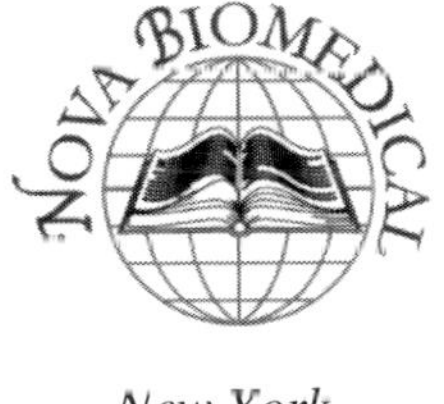

New York

Library of Congress Cataloging-in-Publication Data

Library of Congress Control Number: 2014948642

ISBN: 978-1-63321-859-8

Published by Nova Science Publishers, Inc. † New York

Contents

Preface

Carotid artery disease causes approximately 10 to 20% of strokes, and appropriate intervention is important for secondary and primary stroke prevention. Aggressive treatment of modifiable risk factors for carotid atherosclerosis is central to stroke prevention. This book discusses the risk factors, prognosis and management of carotid artery disease. Topics include medical and behavioral intervention for carotid atherosclerotic disease; intracranial carotid artery stenosis diagnosed with CTA; carotid artery atherosclerosis in patients with inflammatory joint diseases; the impact of obesity on carotid artery disease in obese adolescents; and asymptomatic carotid disease.

Chapter 1 – Carotid artery disease causes approximately 10 to 20% of strokes, and appropriate intervention is important for secondary and primary stroke prevention. Aggressive treatment of modifiable risk factors for carotid atherosclerosis is central to stroke prevention.

Patients with both asymptomatic and symptomatic carotid artery stenosis should be screened for treatable stroke risk factors with implementation of appropriate lifestyle changes (including healthy diet, smoking cessation, physical activity) and medical management. Intensive medical management may be a reasonable alternative to invasive treatment in patients with asymptomatic carotid disease.

Antihypertensive treatment is recommended for patients with hypertension and asymptomatic or symptomatic extracranial carotid atherosclerosis but treatment goals must consider the risk of reduced cerebral perfusion with aggressive treatment, pending correction of stenosis. Lipid lowering therapy with statins reduces the risk of stroke in patients with atherosclerosis and is effective for both primary and secondary stroke prevention leading to stabilization and even regression of intima–media thickness of the carotid-artery wall. Finally, antiplatelet therapy reduces the incidence of stroke in patients at high risk for atherosclerosis (including patients with asymptomatic carotid atherosclerotic disease) and in those with known symptomatic cerebrovascular disease.

Chapter 2 – Background: The prevalence and impact of intracranial atherosclerosis in the white population is sparsely researched and optimal treatment remains to be defined. Previously, the authos found that 84% of the patients with extracranial internal carotid artery (ICA) stenosis also had an intracranial ICA stenosis diagnosed with CT angiography (CTA). The purpose of this chapter is to investigate the relation between intracranial ICA stenosis and outcome.

Methods: The authors conducted a single center cohort study with long-term follow-up of 84 patients with TIA or infarct that underwent a CTA for the assessment of a carotid artery stenosis between April 1, 2006 and December 31, 2008. Intracranial ICA stenosis was categorised in four groups: without any stenosis (<30%), with any stenosis ($\geq$ 30%), without severe stenosis (<70%), and with severe stenosis ($\geq$ 70%), Primary outcome was recurrent TIA or infarct. Secondary outcomes were MI, vascular death and functional outcome. Poor functional outcome was defined as mRS $\geq$3.

Results: Mean follow-up in the 84 patients was 4.1 years ($\pm$1.2 years). Comparing patients without stenosis to patients with any stenosis ($\geq$30%), no differences in primary and secondary outcomes were found. Severe stenosis ($\geq$70%) was not associated with recurrent stroke, but was strongly associated with vascular death (OR 7.85 (1.9 - 32.5)) and poor functional outcome (OR 4.33 (1.15 - 16.37)).

Conclusion: Severe intracranial ICA stenosis on CTA in a white population is associated with a higher rate of vascular death and poor functional outcome.

Chapter 3 – Patients with inflammatory joint diseases (IJD) have an increased risk of cardiovascular (CV) disease, which is of similar magnitude as for patients with diabetes; approximately twice as high as in the general population. Available CV risk calculators for the general population underestimate future CV events in patients with RA. The underestimation of CV risk may have several reasons:

1   systemic inflammation
2   a lipid paradox which has been described for patients with RA, whereby lower total cholesterol and low-density lipoprotein

cholesterol were associated with increased risk of CV morbidity and mortality

3   the high frequency of asymptomatic carotid plaques (CP) in patients with RA.

In the recent European guidelines for CV disease prevention, CP is considered a very high CV disease risk factor; a CV disease equivalent. Therefore, it is recommended to initiate intensive lipid lowering treatment with statins when CP has been identified in a patient. Thus it is important to identify CP.

Chapter 4 – Obesity is a multifactorial disease, characterized by excessive body fat accumulation, which is increasing worldwide in all age. Excessive body fat is related to a chronic inflammation due to the pro-inflammatory adipokines secreted mainly by visceral fat. Additionally, this inflammation is related to cardiometabolic alterations, such as insulin resistance, dyslipidemia, hypertension, hyperleptinemia, metabolic syndrome and non-alcoholic fatty liver disease, which potentiate cardiovascular risks, such as increase in carotid intima media thickness (cIMT), including in adolescence. The present chapter aims to review the role of obesity and its comorbidities on carotid artery disease in obese adolescents, and the main effects of physical exercise and nutrition. Carotid Intima media thickness (cIMT) is considered an important method of estimating early subclinical signal of atherosclerosis process. An increase of carotid artery is a result from endothelial dysfunction that creates lipid deposits in the intima media of systemic arteries. Such deposits can be caused by inflammation, metabolic alterations and saturated fatty acid intake. The exposure during childhood to these metabolic alterations may contribute to the development of atherosclerosis. In obese adolescents, insulin resistance, visceral fat, leptin/adiponectin ratio and PAI-1 concentration were positive associated with cIMT. Additionally, the diet can also influence carotid artery in obese patients. Saturated fatty acids can predict cIMT, and every 10g of saturated fatty intake per day was associated with increase of 0.03 mm on cIMT. On the other hand, interdisciplinary intervention has been effective in reducing cIMT in obese adolescents with comorbidities, such as metabolic syndrome, non-alcoholic fatty liver disease, hyperleptinemia and insulin resistance. Moreover, reduction in 10% of weight loss can contribute in cIMT reduction in obese adolescents. In conclusion, obesity and metabolic disorders appeared to explain increase of carotid artery disorders, enhancing cardiovascular risks. However, interdisciplinary therapy, including nutritional interventions and physical exercise, may prevent and control obesity related comorbidities, associated with a control of increase in cIMT in obese adolescents.

Chapter 5 – Currently, there is a wide discussion about the role of carotid endarterectomy in asymptomatic carotid disease. Current guidelines recommend that it is *"reasonable to perform carotid endarterectomy in asymptomatic patients with >70% internal carotid artery stenosis if the risk of perioperative stroke, myocardial infarction and death is low"*. This recommendation is largely based on two randomized controlled trials of carotid endarterectomy (CEA) which were performed more than a decade ago in patients with asymptomatic carotid stenosis. However, more recent data suggest that perhaps we cannot rely on these trials to guide our clinical practice nowadays. In this context, many scientists underline the need for new trials which are indeed ongoing. Moreover, nowadays there are several imaging techniques available which assist us to identify which carotid plaques are associated with the higher stroke risk.

In: Carotid Artery Disease
Editor: Sherri Derricks

ISBN: 978-1-63321-859-8
© 2014 Nova Science Publishers, Inc.

Chapter 1

Medical and Behavioral Intervention for Carotid Atherosclerotic Disease

Angelos Liontos, MD,
Haralampos Milionis, MD, PhD, FESO and
*George Ntaios, MD, MSc, ESO, PhD, FESO**
Department of Internal Medicine, School of Medicine,
University of Ioannina, Ioannina, Greece

Abstract

Carotid artery disease causes approximately 10 to 20% of strokes, and appropriate intervention is important for secondary and primary stroke prevention. Aggressive treatment of modifiable risk factors for carotid atherosclerosis is central to stroke prevention.

Patients with both asymptomatic and symptomatic carotid artery stenosis should be screened for treatable stroke risk factors with implementation of appropriate lifestyle changes (including healthy diet,

* Corresponding author: George Ntaios MD, MSc (ESO Stroke Medicine), PhD, FESO. Assistant Professor of Internal Medicine, Department of Medicine, Larissa University Hospital, School of Medicine, University of Thessaly, Biopolis 41110, Larissa, Greece. T: +30 241 3502888, f: +30 241 3501557, e-mail: gntaios@med.uth.gr.

smoking cessation, physical activity) and medical management. Intensive medical management may be a reasonable alternative to invasive treatment in patients with asymptomatic carotid disease.

Antihypertensive treatment is recommended for patients with hypertension and asymptomatic or symptomatic extracranial carotid atherosclerosis but treatment goals must consider the risk of reduced cerebral perfusion with aggressive treatment, pending correction of stenosis. Lipid-lowering therapy with statins reduces the risk of stroke in patients with atherosclerosis and is effective for both primary and secondary stroke prevention leading to stabilization and even regression of intima–media thickness of the carotid-artery wall.

Finally, antiplatelet therapy reduces the incidence of stroke in patients at high risk for atherosclerosis (including patients with asymptomatic carotid atherosclerotic disease) and in those with known symptomatic cerebrovascular disease.

Introduction

Carotid artery disease due to atherosclerosis, the most common disease affecting the carotid artery, causes approximately 10 to 20% of strokes and TIAs [1-5]. Intensive and targeted intervention is important for primary and secondary stroke prevention in patients with both asymptomatic and symptomatic carotid stenosis [1]. The degree of carotid stenosis is associated with the stroke risk and along with the presence of symptoms (previous stroke or TIA) are the determinants of the intervention (invasive or not) suggested by current guidelines for the clinicians [1].

Current guidelines from the American Heart Association, American Stroke Association, European Society of Cardiology and the European Stroke Organization for both primary and secondary prevention of stroke in patients with carotid artery disease suggest intensive and aggressive treatment of all the modifiable and treatable risk factors [6-11].

Carotid stenosis is a potentially preventable cause of stroke [2]. In patients with carotid stenosis in either primary or secondary prevention, the appropriate risk factor modification and treatment with the best medical therapy has become a powerful tool for reduction of stroke risk to reduce both early and long-term risks of vascular events, dementia, and death [8, 9, 12, 13].

In the primary prevention of stroke two actions should take place: a) population approach which aims to change all risk factors in the entire population (environmental or lifestyle factors such as diet, physical activity, smoking, and obesity) [14] and b) high-risk strategy which will help at identifying currently asymptomatic individuals at high risk of future vascular disease to reduce their individual risk [15, 16].

It is estimated that through lifestyle interventions 70% of stroke and over 80% of CHD might be preventable [15].

In the primary prevention of carotid stenosis there are no RCTs available for the preventive treatment of patients with arteriosclerotic carotid stenosis. These patients, at increased risk for vascular events, should undergo lifestyle modifications (smoking cessation, normalization of body weight, and adequate exercise) [17].

Pharmacologic therapy helps at reducing the risk for worsening atherosclerosis and reducing the risk of an acute complication of stable disease, such as atherothrombotic stroke or transient ischemic attack [18] and thus medical treatment of arterial hypertension, lipid metabolic disorders, diabetes mellitus and oral anticoagulation with acetylsalicylic acid should be administrated [17].

Intermediate- and long-term secondary prevention corresponds to primary and secondary stroke prophylaxis, especially with respect to risk factor modification and optimal medical treatment [7, 8, 17]. The risk of stroke within 90 days after a TIA is 10-20%, with approximately one-half of these strokes occurring within the first 48 hours after initial presentation [15].

Early initiation of treatment after a TIA, including medication and surgical intervention, can significantly reduce the risk of early stroke [15].

Behavioral Intervention

Lifestyle factors such as a healthy diet, physical activity, abstinence from smoking, moderate alcohol intake and maintenance of a 'healthy" body weight reduces the risk of cardiovascular disease and mortality [10]. A sedentary lifestyle is associated with increased risk of stroke [8].

Although patients are aware of the presence of carotid artery stenosis as a risk factor of stroke and the need to modify lifestyle habits is now established it does not seem to lead to improved health behaviors [18].

Although lifestyle habits have an important impact on post-stroke outcomes, there are no published trials of lifestyle interventions for secondary stroke prevention [10]. There is little evidence about sex differences in the effect of healthy lifestyle on stroke prevalence and outcomes and further research is needed to develop lifestyle interventions that are effective for both primary and secondary stroke prevention in men and women [10].

There are not any particular recommendations regarding patients with carotid atherosclerosis. However, interventions in lifestyle changes should be considered as in all patients at risk of stroke [10, 15, 18]. Of note, in current recommendations, there is a special focus to non-optimal diet is contributing in the pathogenesis of high blood pressure which is the major modifiable risk factor for ischemic stroke (and/or carotid atherosclerosis) through excess salt intake, low potassium intake, excess weight, high alcohol consumption [8, 19].

Physical Activity

Physical inactivity is an important risk factor for the development of vascular disease [20] and increased risk of total mortality, cardiovascular mortality, cardiovascular morbidity and stroke [8].

Large prospective cohort studies and meta-analyses have shown that higher levels of physical activity reduce all-cause mortality [21] and cardiovascular mortality [8, 22-24]. The effect of physical activity is through reducing BP [25] and controlling other risk factors for CVD [26], including diabetes, [25] and excess body weight [8], enhance vasodilation [27], improve glucose tolerance, [28] and promote cardiovascular health [7, 29].

Other biological mechanisms are the reduction in plasma fibrinogen and platelet activity and the elevation in plasma tissue plasminogen activator activity and HDL-cholesterol concentrations [8, 30-32].

Physical inactivity is a modifiable risk factor for stroke, has a beneficial effect on multiple stroke risk factors, including carotid athrerosclerotic disease [7, 29, 33, 34]. The risk reduction of stroke associated with the physical activity is unknown [35, 36] and few studies have examined its role on stroke mortality [8].

The relationship between physical activity and carotid IMT as a marker of subclinical atherosclerosis has not always been consistent [37-39] and is not clear whether exercise alone is beneficial to stroke risk reduction [35].

Tobacco Smoking

Smoking increases blood pressure and contributes to the progression of atherosclerosis [15] and there is a dose-depended relationship between smoking and cerebral ischemia, with the heaviest smokers at the highest risk [7, 15].

It also leads to an increased risk for silent brain infarction and as shown in the Cardiovascular Health Study, smoking was associated with a substantially increased risk for stroke recurrence in the elderly [9].

In large epidemiological studies, cigarette smoking has been associated with extracranial carotid artery IMT and the severity of carotid artery stenosis [40-43].

In the ARIC study it was shown that tobacco use increases the progression of carotid IMT over 3 years compared with nonsmokers, in both current and past users (50% and 25% respectively) [35, 44]. The Framingham Heart Study showed that extracranial carotid artery stenosis correlated with the quantity of cigarettes smoked over time [35, 45] and in the Cardiovascular Health Study the severity of carotid artery stenosis was greater in current smokers than in former smokers [35]. There was a significant relationship between the severity of carotid stenosis and pack-years of tobacco use [35, 46].

In the NOMASS and the BCID (Berlin Cerebral Ischemia Databank) studies, respectively, the RRs of >60% carotid stenosis were 1.5 and 3.9 among cigarette smokers with cerebral ischemia [35].

All smokers with carotid atherosclerosis should be advised to quit and should be offered smoking cessation interventions.

Obesity and the Metabolic Syndrome

The metabolic syndrome and abdominal obesity are associated to atherosclerosis and stroke [47, 48]. The metabolic syndrome is defined by the World Health Organization and the National Cholesterol Education Program on the basis of blood glucose, hypertension, dyslipidemia, body mass index, waist/hip ratio, and urinary albumin excretion [35]. The NCEP Adult Treatment Panel III (ATP III) defined metabolic syndrome as the presence of ≥ 3 of the following criteria: (1) abdominal obesity as determined by waist circumference >102 cm (or >40 inches) for men and >88 cm or (>35 inches) for women; (2) triglycerides ≥ 150 mg/dL, (3) HDL cholesterol <40 mg/dL for men and <50 mg/dL for women, (4) BP $\geq 130/\geq 85$ mm Hg; and (5) fasting glucose ≥ 110 mg/dL [49]. The International Diabetes Foundation (IDF) modified the definition proposing waist circumference >88 cm for men and >80 cm in women plus 2 of the other NCEP-ATP III criteria. Obesity and unhealthy lifestyle in addition to other genetic and acquired factors seem to interact to produce the metabolic syndrome [8]. AHA and several other organizations proposed a definition that requires any 3 of the following criteria: waist circumference (population and country-specific cutoffs), plasma triglyceride ≥150 mg/dL (1.7 mmol/L), HDL-cholesterol <40 mg/dL (1.0 mmol/L) for men or <50 mg/dL (1.3 mmol/L) for women, blood pressure ≥130mm Hg systolic or ≥85 mm Hg diastolic, or fasting glucose ≥100mg/dL (5.6 mmol/L) [9]. Recent research has expanded the syndrome to include subclinical inflammation, disorders of thrombosis/fibrinolysis, and endothelial dysfunction [9].

Metabolic syndrome is highly prevalent with about 22% of adults aged >20 years while among patients with ischemic stroke, the prevalence is 30% to 50% [9]. Data from the National Health and Nutrition Examination Survey, among 10,357 subjects, showed that the prevalence of metabolic syndrome was higher in persons with history of stroke (43.5%) than in subjects with no history of cardiovascular disease (22.8%; $P \leq 0.001$) while it was independently associated with stroke history in all ethnic groups and both sexes (OR, 2.16; 95% CI, 0.48 to 3.16) [8]. The visceral adiposity in the metabolic syndrome is associated with insulin resistance (strongly related to an increased risk for DM) which is an important marker of the metabolic syndrome with many studies showing a relationship between glucose intolerance and stroke risk [8].

Metabolic syndrome is associated with carotid atherosclerosis after adjustment for other risk factors in men and women across several age and ethnic groups [35, 50-52]. This relationship to carotid atherosclerosis is strengthened in proportion to the number of components of metabolic syndrome present ($P<0.001$) [35, 53-55]. with hypertension being the most related risk factor [35, 53-57]. Lipid disorders associated with the metabolic syndrome (hypertriglyceridemia, low HDL-C) and obesity are also related to carotid atherosclerosis in several reports [35, 51]. Behavioral changes and drug therapy to globally modify the features of the metabolic syndrome may be of value in order to reduce the associated risk [9].

Medical Management

Diabetes Mellitus and Other Disorders of Glucose Metabolism

Glucose metabolism disorders are associated with an increased risk of ischemic stroke [9] Impaired fasting glucose (IFG) in the upper limit (fasting glucose 110–125 mg/dL) offers a greater risk of stroke. Impaired glucose tolerance (IGT) and glycated hemoglobin (HbA1c) values from 6.0%-6.5% increase the risk for stroke more than IFG because IGT is a more severe metabolic disorder and elevated HbA1c is a more comprehensive marker of hyperglycemic state than IFG [9].

DM is associated with an increased risk for first ischemic stroke (adjusted RR, 1.5-3) and may be responsible for >8% of first ischemic strokes [9] and this risk of ischemic stroke in patients with diabetes mellitus is increased 2- to 5-fold compared with patients without diabetes [15, 35].

Disorders of glucose metabolism are also highly prevalent among patients who had already a stroke. A 28% of patients with ischemic stroke have pre-diabetes mellitus (DM), and 25-45% have DM [9] in an overall of 60-70% of patients that may have 1 of these dysglycemic states.

The effect of pre-DM on prognosis has not been adequately studied, but DM is associated with increased risk for recurrent ischemic stroke [9] as shown in a substudy of the Cardiovascular Health Study that enrolled patients with a first ischemic stroke; DM was associated with a 60% increased risk for recurrence (RR, 1.59; 95% CI, 1.07–2.37) [9].

DM was also associated with carotid artery stenosis in the Cardiovascular Health Study. The study reported that elevated fasting and post-challenge glucose levels were associated with an increased risk of stroke [58], and DM was associated with carotid IMT and the severity of carotid artery stenosis [35, 59]. In the Insulin Resistance Atherosclerosis Study, diabetes and fasting glucose levels were associated with carotid IMT, and carotid IMT progressed twice more rapidly in patients with diabetes than in those without diabetes [35, 60, 61].

Similarly, in the ARIC study, diabetes was associated with progression of carotid IMT [62, 63] and in the Rotterdam study, diabetes predicted progression to severe carotid obstruction [35].

Among therapeutic interventions for DM, pioglitazone has been reported to cause less progression or induced regression of carotid IMT compared with glimepiride in several randomized studies [35, 64, 65] and intensive insulin therapy the EDIC (Epidemiology of Diabetes Interventions and Complications) study, slowed the progression of carotid IMT which was greater in patients with diabetes than in those without diabetes [66].

No major trials for secondary prevention of stroke have specifically examined interventions for pre-DM or DM. Management of stroke patients with these conditions is based on trials in nonstroke or mixed populations [9].

In most patients who have had a TIA, the A1C target is less than 7% [7, 67] and a more intensive A1C reduction <6% has not been shown to decrease cardiovascular deaths or all-cause mortality [68].

Some studies have suggested, although no drug has been proven to have a direct effect on macrovascular outcomes (including stroke), that tight glycemic control should be targeted [15, 47, 69].

Arterial Hypertension

Hypertension remains one of the most important preventable factors leading to disease and death and is the most common condition in primary care which leads to cardiovascular events, including stroke [70, 71].

Data from population-based studies have shown a clear relationship between hypertension and increased stroke risk which is continuous; the higher the blood pressure, the greater the risk of stroke [8, 12, 15, 47].

With each 10 mmHg increase in systolic blood pressure the risk of stroke rises by 30-45% [12, 15, 47].

Antihypertensive therapy has been shown to reduce the risk of both first and recurrent ischemic stroke [18]. Blood pressure control after a TIA is associated with a 30-40% RR reduction with larger blood pressure decreases resulting to a greater decrease in stroke risk [15, 72, 73]. The protective effect of blood pressure lowering extends even to patients without hypertension, as shown in the HOPE (Heart Outcomes Protection Evaluation) trial, in which patients with systemic atherosclerosis randomized to treatment with ramipril displayed a significantly lower risk of stroke than those given a placebo (relative risk, RR 0.68; $P<0.001$) [35, 74].

Epidemiological studies, including the ARIC study [75], the Cardiovascular Health Study, Framingham Heart Study [45], and MESA (Multi-Ethnic Study of Atherosclerosis), among others, demonstrated a relationship between hypertension and the risk of developing carotid atherosclerosis [18, 35, 46, 75]. In the Framingham Heart Study, there was a 2-fold greater risk of carotid stenosis >25% for each 20-mm Hg increase in systolic blood pressure [45]. In SHEP (Systolic Hypertension in the Elderly Program), systolic blood pressure ≥160 mm Hg was the strongest independent predictor of carotid stenosis [35].

The AHA/ASA guidelines suggest antihypertensive therapy in patients with hypertension and asymptomatic carotid stenosis to maintain a BP below 140/90 mmHg [12].

In symptomatic patients with severe carotid artery stenosis, however, it is unknown whether antihypertensive therapy is beneficial or harmful by reducing cerebral perfusion [35].

It is also suggested that lifestyle modifications associated with blood pressure reduction should be considered including decreasing dietary sodium intake; losing weight; eating a diet rich in fruits, vegetables, and low-fat dairy products; exercising regularly; and consuming alcohol only in moderation [9, 15, 73].

Dyslipidemia

Epidemiological studies have consistently found an association between cholesterol and carotid artery atherosclerosis as determined by measurement of IMT [8, 42, 76, 77]. In the Framingham Heart Study, the RR of carotid artery stenosis >25% was approximately 1.1 for every 10-mg/dL increase in total cholesterol [45] and in the MESA study, carotid plaque lipid core detected by MRI was strongly associated with total cholesterol [35].

Treatment with statins reduces the risk of stroke in patients with atherosclerosis or at high risk for atherosclerosis [8, 35, 78]. The beneficial effect of statins on ischemic stroke is most likely related to their capacity to reduce progression or induce regression of atherosclerosis [8]. The mechanism of stroke protection by statins is not entirely clear. Cholesterol-independent pleiotropic effects may contribute to it: statins reduce inflammation, are anti-atherogenic, lower blood pressure, stabilize plaques, are anti-thrombotic, improve fibrinolysis, and decrease platelet activation. They also have immuno-modulatory effects, increase the number of circulating endothelial progenitor cells, and improve endothelium function [79].

In addition, statins have neuroprotective properties, reduce ischaemic lesion size in animal stroke models, and may therefore also improve stroke outcome [79]. However, the relative contribution of LDL cholesterol lowering vs. other pleiotropic statin actions on the reduction of stroke risk cannot be easily differentiated since essentially all pleiotropic effects of statins are also dependent on HMG-CoA reductase inhibition.

Thus, these effects go hand in hand with any effect on LDL cholesterol levels, are dose-dependent, and correspond with the potency of a given statin drug. In other words, LDL cholesterol may as well serve as a biomarker for pleiotropic statin effects. It is therefore not surprising that there is a linear association between reduction in LDL cholesterol concentration and stroke incidence among the major statin trials [71, 80].

Statins has been shown to reduce the risk of adverse cardiovascular events including ischemic stroke in primary prevention studies [18]. In addition, imaging studies have demonstrated regression of carotid lesions and attenuation of progression of carotid intimal thickening with statin therapy [18]. Overall statins have an excellent tolerability and safety profile [18].

A meta-analysis of statin trials found that LDL-cholesterol reduction correlated inversely with progression of carotid IMT [80]. The beneficial effects on carotid IMT appear to be greater with higher-intensity statin therapy [8, 35, 81-83].

The SPARCL (Stroke Prevention by Aggressive Reduction in Cholesterol Levels) trial prospectively compared the effect of atorvastatin (80 mg daily) against placebo on the risk of stroke among patients with recent stroke or TIA [84]. Statin therapy reduced the absolute risk of stroke at 5 years by 2.2%, the RR of all stroke by 16%, and the RR of ischemic stroke by 22% [35]. Lipid lowering with high-dose atorvastatin reduced the risk of cerebrovascular events in patients with and without carotid stenosis, yet those with carotid stenosis derived greater benefit [35, 85].

Moreover, statin therapy reduced progression or induced regression of carotid atherosclerosis and the subsequent carotid revascularization was reduced by 56% (hazard ratio, HR 0.44, 95% CI 0.24 to 0.79; P=0.006) in the group of atorvastatin [35, 85]. Among 1007 patients with carotid artery stenosis enrolled in the trial, the benefit of statin therapy resulted in a 33% reduction of stroke and a 56% reduction of carotid revascularization procedures at 5 years [11, 85].

In the Heart Protection Study, there was also found a 50% reduction in carotid endarterectomy (CEA) rates in patients randomized to statin therapy [35, 86].

In a meta-analysis of 9 trials of patients randomized to statin treatment or control it was found that for each 10% reduction in LDL cholesterol the risk of all strokes reduced by 15.6% (95% CI 6.7 to 23.6) and of carotid IMT reduced by 0.73% per year (95% CI 0.27 to 1.19) [35, 80].

In METEOR (Measuring Effects on Intima-Media Thickness: An Evaluation of Rosuvastatin), rosuvastatin treatment compared with placebo reduced progression of carotid IMT over 2 years in patients with low Framingham risk scores and elevated serum LDL cholesterol levels [35, 81].

In the ARBITER (Arterial Biology for the Investigation of the Treatment Effects of Reducing Cholesterol) trial, carotid IMT regressed after 12 months of treatment with atorvastatin (80 mg daily) but remained unchanged after treatment with pravastatin (40 mg daily) [83].

The corresponding LDL cholesterol levels were and were 76±23 in the atorvastatin group vs. 110±30 mg/dL in the pravastatin treatment group [35, 83].

In the ASAP (Atorvastatin versus Simvastatin on Atherosclerosis Progression) trial of patients with familial hypercholesterolemia, carotid IMT decreased after 2 years of treatment with 80 mg of atorvastatin daily but increased in patients randomized to 40 mg of simvastatin daily [35, 82].

The effect of lipid lowering therapies other than statins on the risk of ischemic stroke or the severity of carotid artery disease is not established [35].

Another combination of lipid lowering agents, i.e. colestipol and niacin, reduced progression of carotid IMT [35, 87].

In the ARBITER-2 study of patients with carotid disease and low levels of HDL cholesterol, carotid IMT progression did not differ significantly after the addition of extended-release niacin to statin therapy compared with statin therapy alone, although there was a trend favoring the dual therapy [35, 88]. However, in the ENHANCE (Effect of Combination Ezetimibe and High-Dose Simvastatin vs. Simvastatin Alone on the Atherosclerotic Process in Patients with Heterozygous Familial Hypercholesterolemia) study, in patients with familial hypercholesterolemia, the addition of ezetimibe to simvastatin did not affect progression of carotid IMT more than the use of simvastatin alone [35].

Current European Guidelines recommend the use of statins in patients with established atherosclerosis, including carotid artery disease to a goal of LDL cholesterol <100 mg/dL. In patients with diabetes mellitus and carotid atherosclerosis the recommended LDL goal is below 70 mg/dL [18]. It is also recommended that if treatment with a statin does not achieve the LDL goal, additional drug therapy (e.g. bile acid sequestrants or niacin) should be considered while patients who cannot take statin therapy should be given alternative LDL lowering drugs [18].

Antithrombotic Therapy

Antiplatelet Therapy

Antiplatelet drugs reduce the risk of stroke compared with placebo in patients with TIA or previous stroke [89] and is a mainstay in the treatment of symptomatic carotid disease but no adequately powered controlled studies have shown the efficacy of platelet-inhibitor drugs for prevention of stroke in asymptomatic patients with carotid atherosclerotic disease [35].

In 23,748 patients with acute ischaemic stroke of presumed arterial origin, anticoagulation started within 48 h of stroke reduced early recurrent ischaemic stroke (OR 0·76, 95% CI 0·65–0·88) but increased symptomatic intracranial haemorrhage (2·55, 1·95–3·33), and achieved no net benefit in reducing any recurrent stroke (0·97, 0·85–1·11) [13, 90].

In patients with carotid stenosis undergoing either primary or secondary prevention, aspirin and the combination of aspirin and extended released dipyridamole, clopidogrel, ticlopidine, and triflusal have been shown to be effective [2]. Currently, aspirin, aspirin/extended dipyridamole, or clopidogrel is used in clinical practice [2].

Aspirin

Current data support the use of aspirin in patients with asymptomatic carotid artery disease and aspirin therapy is considered be beneficial in high-risk patients with carotid artery stenosis, and is also recommended for patients with obstructive atherosclerosis involving the carotid artery. [18] Treatment with aspirin (ASA) after ischemic stroke or TIA lends a 23% risk reduction of subsequent non-fatal stroke [12]. The use of low-dose aspirin (75–150 mg daily) is well established in the prevention of stroke and is used routinely in the management of CAD [47].

Guidelines recommend aspirin at a dose between 75 and 325 mg daily. In general, low dose aspirin (75–81 mg) has been shown to be as effective as higher doses in high-risk patients [18].

The Asymptomatic Cervical Bruit Study compared aspirin 325 mg daily, against placebo in asymptomatic patients with carotid stenosis of >50%. After 2 years of follow-up, the annual rate of ischemic events and death due to any cause was 12.3% in the placebo group and 11.0% in the aspirin group (P=0.61). In the Veterans Affairs Cooperative Study Group [91] and ACAS, [92] the stroke rates were approximately 2% per year in groups treated with aspirin alone [35, 91-93].

Aspirin also reduces the risk of recurrent stroke and other major vascular events by about 13% compared with control [13]. As single antiplatelet therapy, aspirin 160–300 mg daily, started within 48 h of onset of ischaemic stroke in 40,000 patients, and continued for 2–4 weeks, reduced the odds of recurrent ischaemic stroke by 23% (2·4% aspirin *vs* 3·1% control; odds ratio [OR] 0·77, 95% CI 0·69–0·87), increased the odds of symptomatic intracranial haemorrhage by 22% (1·0% *vs* 0·8%; OR 1·22, 95% CI 1·00–1·50), and reduced the odds of any recurrent stroke by 12% (3·4% *vs* 3·9%; OR 0·88, 95% CI 0·79–0·97) compared with control [13] Doses >150 mg/day are associated with more side effects [2, 94].

In the Antithrombotic Trialists' Collaboration, a meta-analysis of >60 aspirin trials, the best risk reduction was found in trials using a 75-to-150 mg dose of aspirin [95-97]. In patients with a history of aspirin-induced ulcer bleeding, aspirin in combination with a proton-pump inhibitor was superior to clopidogrel alone in the prevention of recurrent ulcer bleeding [2, 98].

Randomized studies have compared aspirin with CEA in symptomatic patients with carotid stenosis [99]. In NASCET, patients with >70% stenosis had a stroke rate of 24% after 18 months, and those with 50% to 69% stenosis had a stroke rate of 22% over 5 years with antiplatelet therapy (predominantly aspirin) and without revascularization [35, 100].

The data regarding antiplatelet regimens in patients receiving CEA or carotid artery stenting (CAS) is less robust than that for overall secondary stroke prevention. Low dose aspirin (75 mg) reduces the number of perioperative stroke, in patients receiving CEA, without increasing bleeding risk [12]. In the randomized double blind Acetylsalicylic Acid and Carotid Endarterectomy (ACE) study low dose aspirin (81 or 325 mg) was superior to high dose aspirin (650 mg or 1300 mg) in reduction of a combined endpoint of stroke, MI, and death at both 30 days (5.4 vs. 7.0 %, P<0.07) and 3 months (6.2 vs. 8.4 %, P<0.03) [12].

Aspirin vs. Clopidogrel

Clopidogrel monotherapy has been shown to be beneficial compared to aspirin for secondary prevention in patients with established carotid disease; however, patients with asymptomatic carotid disease alone were not studied [18].

Dual Antiplatelet Therapy

Trials evaluating dual antiplatelet therapy with aspirin and a thienopyridine compared to aspirin alone in stable patients with atherosclerotic vascular disease or risk factors have not shown benefit [18]. Dual antiplatelet therapy (DAPT) in patients with recent TIA or stroke was initially investigated in the Management of Atherothrombosis with Clopidogrel in High-risk Patients (MATCH) trial [12]. In the MATCH and CHARISMA (Clopidogrel for High Atherothrombotic Risk and Ischemic Stabilization, Management, and Avoidance) trials, the combination of clopidogrel and aspirin did not reduce stroke risk compared with either treatment alone [101, 102].

In the CHARISMA trial compared aspirin and clopidogrel against aspirin alone in both symptomatic and asymptomatic patients with carotid disease, analysis showed that the rate of primary event of stroke was similar in both groups (6.8% vs 7.3%; P = .22) [2, 20, 101].

The Clopidogrel and Aspirin for Reduction of Emboli in Symptomatic Carotid Stenosis (CARESS) trial showed that in patients with recently symptomatic carotid stenosis combination therapy with clopidogrel and aspirin is more effective than aspirin alone in reducing asymptomatic embolization in a short-term followup [2]. The optimal perioperative treatment of patients with carotid stenosis, on dual antiplatelet therapy (DAPT) with aspirin and clopidogrel remains unclear. A randomized trial by Payne et al. evaluated the effect of clopidogrel therapy in combination with aspirin in decreasing the burden of postoperative embolization [12].

The DAPT group had a significant decrease in the magnitude of embolization as measured by transcranial Doppler (2.2 vs. 18.5%) [12]. DAPT should be continued for at least 1 month after carotid stent placement and ideally for 3 months considering stent endothelialization is a prolonged process, taking between 28-96 days [12]. Long-term aspirin plus clopidogrel is not more effective than either aspirin alone (RR 0·89, 95% CI 0·78–1·01) or clopidogrel alone (1·01, 0·93–1·08) in preventing recurrent stroke, and causes more intracranial haemorrhage than clopidogrel alone (1·46, 1·17–1·82) but not aspirin alone (0·99, 0·70–1·42) [13, 101-103].

Cilostazol

Cilostazol, a phosphodiesterase III inhibitor, has shown to be an antiplatelet, vasodilatory, and antithrombotic agent. In patients of Asian descent, cilostazol 100 mg twice daily reduces recurrent ischaemic stroke by 19 % (RR 0·81, 95% CI 0·62–1·06, I^2=0%), haemorrhagic stroke by 73% (RR 0·27, 95% CI 0·13–0·54, I^2=0%), and major vascular events by 28% (RR 0·72, 95% CI 0·57–0·89, I^2=0%) compared with aspirin [13, 104].

One case series looked at 207 patients who had been given cilostazol after carotid artery stenting (CAS). Cilostazol seemed to reduce the incidence of restenosis, target vessel revascularization, hemorrhage, death, or thromboembolism (15.0% vs 19.9%; log-rank, P = .17) [105].

Another study assessed the impact of cilostazol on carotid artery plaques after carotid endarectomy. Thirty-four patients were given cilostazol while the remaining 48 patients were given aspirin (n = 33), ticlopidine (n = 8), clopidogrel (n = 2), or warfarin (n = 5). Patients were assessed by measuring intimal thickness using ultrasound for up to 6 years. There was no evidence of ipslateral or contralateral plaque development in any of the patients taking cilostazol. In the second group, seven patients were found to have evidence of restenosis in the ipslateral or plaque formation in the contralateral artery. Interestingly, six out of the seven of these patients had hyperlipidemia. This shows that there is a promising role in carotid artery stenosis, but higher-powered randomized trials need to be conducted to establish its true effect [20].

Anticoagulant Therapy

Anticoagulants have often been used as an alternative to antiplatelets in patients with ischemic strokes [20]. Vitamin K antagonists at any dose are not more effective than antiplatelet therapy in reducing recurrent stroke (medium intensity anticoagulation: RR 0·80, 95% CI 0·56–1·14; high intensity anticoagulation: RR 1·02, 95% CI 0·49–2·13) in patients with ischaemic stroke or TIA caused by presumed arterial disease, but cause more major haemorrhage [13, 106]. The WARSS (Warfarin-Aspirin Recurrent Stroke Study) compared aspirin and warfarin for stroke prevention in patients with recent stroke [107]. In the subgroup with severe large-artery stenosis or occlusion (259 patients), including carotid atherosclerosis, there was no benefit of warfarin over aspirin after 2 years [35]. It is recommended that anticoagulation in patients with carotid stenosis should not be used after noncardioembolic ischemic strokes since high-intensity anticoagulation (INR 3.0–4.5) is more hazardous than effective compared to antiplatelet therapy [2].

Data for patients with carotid artery stenosis and the novel oral anticoagulants is lacking, and therefore, it is difficult to suggest its use in patients who have had a stroke as a result of carotid artery stenosis [20].

Hyperhomocysteinemia

Homocysteine is an amino acid that is derived from the metabolism of the essential amino acid methionine [108]. Increased plasma levels of homocysteine are often a consequence of reduced enzymatic activity in its metabolic pathways [109]. Occasionally, drugs may interfere with homocysteine levels [110]. The prevalence of elevated levels of homocysteine is common in healthy men (43%) and women (47%) aged ≥60 years [9] and about 75% of the cases of high homocysteine levels are associated with low folate or vitamin B12 concentrations [9]. Hyperhomocysteinemia increases the risk of stroke [35]. Cohort and case-control studies have shown a 2-fold greater risk of stroke associated with hyperhomocysteinemia [9]. A meta-analysis of 30 studies, enrolling more than 16 000 patients, found a 25% difference in plasma homocysteine concentration (3 micromoles/lt), to be associated with a 19% difference in stroke risk [35, 89]. The VISP (Vitamin Intervention for Stroke Prevention) study showed that 70% of patients with a noncardioembolic stroke have mild to moderate hyperhomocysteinemia [9]. In the other hand in patients <45 years with arterial occlusive disease, moderate hyperhomocysteinemia was found in 19.2% (95% CI, 9.0%–31.9%) [9].

The risk of developing >25% extracranial carotid stenosis is increased 2-fold among elderly patients with elevated homocysteine levels while plasma concentrations of folate and pyridoxal 5′ phosphate are inversely associated with carotid stenosis [35]. Carotid IMT and carotid artery stenosis are increased in persons with elevated homocysteine levels [8].

In the ARIC study, increased carotid IMT was 3-fold more likely among individuals with the highest than the lowest quintile of homocysteine [35, 111]. In the Study of Health Assessment and Risk in Ethnic groups (SHARE), a cross-sectional study of south Asian Chinese and white Canadians, plasma homocysteine >11.7 μmol/L was associated with increased carotid IMT [8]. It has to be noted though that several recent investigations found that the relationship between homocysteine levels and carotid IMT was eliminated after adjustment for other cardiovascular risk factors or renal function [8, 112].

Most studies of patients with established atherosclerotic vascular disease have found no benefit of homocysteine lowering by B-complex vitamin therapy on surrogate endpoints [113-115] or clinical cardiovascular end points [8]. The B-complex vitamins pyridoxine (B_6), cobalamin (B_{12}), and folic acid lower homocysteine levels. In a clinical trial of healthy adults without diabetes and CVD it was shown that B-complex vitamin supplementation compared with placebo decreased carotid IMT in the group of participants whose baseline plasma homocysteine was ≥9.1 μmol/L, but not in those whose homocysteine levels were lower [8, 116].

A substudy of the Vitamins to Prevent Stroke (VITATOPS) trial reported that B-complex vitamins did not reduce the change in carotid IMT [112] while in the Atherosclerosis and Folic Acid Supplementation Trial (ASFAST) folic acid did not significantly affect carotid IMT [8, 117].

In patients with carotid disease, hyperhomocysteinemia is a marker of risk but not a target for treatment, and vitamin supplementation does not appear to affect clinical outcomes. Current guidelines consider the evidence insufficient to justify a recommendation for or against routine therapeutic use of vitamin supplements in patients with carotid stenosis [35].

Elevated Lipoprotein(A) Levels

Lipoprotein(a) [Lp(a)] is a low-density lipoprotein particle. In this particle the apolipoprotein B-100 is linked to the glycoprotein apoprotein(a) and it has similar structure and chemical properties to low-density lipoprotein (LDL) [8].

Apoprotein(a) due to its structural homology to plasminogen inhibits fibrinolysis binding to the catalytic complex of plasminogen, tissue plasminogen activator, and fibrin and thus contributing to thrombosis [8].

In experimental models Lp(a) contributes to atherogenesis and is associated with an increased risk for coronary artery disease [8].

Some population-based epidemiological studies have found that Lp(a) is associated with an increased risk of stroke [8, 118].

Several studies have found that Lp(a) level is associated with the severity of carotid artery stenosis and occlusion [8, 119]. In one study higher Lp(a) levels were associated with large-vessel atherothrombotic disease causing stroke, comparing to levels in patients with lacunar stroke [8].

The use of niacin might be reasonable for prevention of ischemic stroke in patients with high Lp(a), but its effectiveness is not well established (Class IIb; Level of Evidence B) [8].

Inflammation

Several inflammatory conditions and markers are associated with stroke risk. Inflammation affects the initiation, growth, and destabilization of atherosclerotic lesions [8]. A number of serum markers of inflammation, including fibrinogen, serum amyloid A, interleukin 6 and high-sensitivity C-reactive protein (hs-CRP) have been proposed as risk markers [8, 120].

Nevertheless, monitoring of all markers of inflammation for population screening is not suggested [8]. The role of inflammation as a risk factor for stroke can be assessed by the examination of the incidence of vascular disease in persons with systemic chronic inflammatory diseases, such as rheumatoid arthritis (RA) and systemic lupus erythematosus (SLE) [8].

In many prospective cohort studies it has been shown an increased risks for cardiovascular disease (including stroke) in persons with RA (odds ratios 1.4-2.0) compared with persons without RA [8]. Women with RA between 35-55 years old were at higher risk [8]. Even though stroke rates were not assessed in patients with SLE, several studies have shown a higher prevalence of atherosclerotic plaque in the carotid arteries of patients with RA or SLE compared with control subjects [121-123] while these patients might be considered a subgroup at high risk for CVD [8].

Risk Factor Modification in Patients Receiving Invasive Treatment

Current guidelines suggest: optimal medical therapy, which should include antiplatelet therapy, statin therapy, and risk factor modification, is recommended for all patients with carotid artery stenosis and a TIA or stroke (*Class I; Level of Evidence A*) in addition to invasive treatment [9].

Randomized trials have demonstrated benefit for carotid endarterectomy (CEA) in appropriately selected patients compared to medical therapy alone. The benefit, in asymptomatic patients is less than that seen in symptomatic patients. Multispecialty guidelines suggest that it is reasonable for patients with a 70% stenosis of the internal carotid artery to undergo CEA if the risk of adverse perioperative events is low [18].

All patients undergoing CEA should receive perioperative medical management according to proper cardiovascular risk assessment. Low-dose aspirin is efficacious to reduce perioperative stroke [95, 124, 125]. There is no clear benefit of dual therapy or high-dose antiplatelet therapy in patients undergoing CEA [11]. The benefit of perioperative statin therapy also is evident in patients receiving CEA [12].

References

[1]   Grotta, J. C. Clinical practice. Carotid stenosis. *The New England journal of medicine*. 2013;369:1143-1150.

[2]   Lovrencic-Huzjan, A., Rundek, T., Katsnelson, M. Recommendations for management of patients with carotid stenosis. *Stroke research and treatment*. 2012;2012:175869.

[3]   Michel, P., Odier, C., Rutgers, M., Reichhart, M., Maeder, P., Meuli, R., et al. The acute stroke registry and analysis of lausanne (astral): Design and baseline analysis of an ischemic stroke registry including acute multimodal imaging. *Stroke; a journal of cerebral circulation*. 2010;41: 2491-2498.

[4]	Ntaios, G., Michel, P. Temporal distribution and magnitude of the vulnerability period around stroke depend on stroke subtype. *Cerebrovascular diseases.* 2011;32:246-253.

[5]	Ntaios, G., Papavasileiou, V., Makaritsis, K., Milionis, H., Michel, P., Vemmos, K. Association of ischaemic stroke subtype with long-term cardiovascular events. *European journal of neurology: the official journal of the European Federation of Neurological Societies.* 2014.

[6]	Brott, T. G., Halperin, J. L., Abbara, S., Bacharach, J. M., Barr, J. D., Bush, R. L., et al. 2011 asa/accf/aha/aann/aans/acr/asnr/cns/saip/scai/sir/snis/svm/svs guideline on the management of patients with extracranial carotid and vertebral artery disease: Executive summary: A report of the american college of cardiology foundation/american heart association task force on practice guidelines, and the american stroke association, american association of neuroscience nurses, american association of neurological surgeons, american college of radiology, american society of neuroradiology, congress of neurological surgeons, society of atherosclerosis imaging and prevention, society for cardiovascular angiography and interventions, society of interventional radiology, society of neurointerventional surgery, society for vascular medicine, and society for vascular surgery. Developed in collaboration with the american academy of neurology and society of cardiovascular computed tomography. *Catheterization and cardiovascular interventions: official journal of the Society for Cardiac Angiography and Interventions.* 2013;81:E76-123.

[7]	Furie, K. L., Kasner, S. E., Adams, R. J., Albers, G. W., Bush, R. L., Fagan, S. C., et al. Guidelines for the prevention of stroke in patients with stroke or transient ischemic attack: A guideline for healthcare professionals from the american heart association/american stroke association. *Stroke; a journal of cerebral circulation.* 2011;42:227-276.

[8]	Goldstein, L. B., Bushnell, C. D., Adams, R. J., Appel, L. J., Braun, L. T., Chaturvedi, S., et al. Guidelines for the primary prevention of stroke: A guideline for healthcare professionals from the american heart association/american stroke association. *Stroke; a journal of cerebral circulation.* 2011;42:517-584.

[9]	Kernan, W. N., Ovbiagele, B., Black, H. R., Bravata, D. M., Chimowitz, M. I., Ezekowitz, M. D., et al. Guidelines for the prevention of stroke in patients with stroke and transient ischemic attack: A guideline for healthcare professionals from the american heart association/american stroke association. *Stroke; a journal of cerebral circulation.* 2014.

[10] Bushnell, C., McCullough, L. D., Awad, I. A., Chireau, M. V., Fedder, W. N., Furie, K. L., et al. Guidelines for the prevention of stroke in women: A statement for healthcare professionals from the american heart association/american stroke association. *Stroke; a journal of cerebral circulation.* 2014;45:1545-1588.

[11] European Stroke, O., Tendera, M., Aboyans, V., Bartelink, M. L., Baumgartner, I., Clement, D., et al. Esc guidelines on the diagnosis and treatment of peripheral artery diseases: Document covering atherosclerotic disease of extracranial carotid and vertebral, mesenteric, renal, upper and lower extremity arteries: The task force on the diagnosis and treatment of peripheral artery diseases of the european society of cardiology (esc). *European heart journal.* 2011;32:2851-2906.

[12] Litsky, J., Stilp, E., Njoh, R., Mena-Hurtado, C. Management of symptomatic carotid disease in 2014. *Current cardiology reports.* 2014; 16:462.

[13] Hankey, G. J. Secondary stroke prevention. *Lancet neurology.* 2014;13: 178-194.

[14] Lopez, A. D., Mathers, C. D., Ezzati, M., Jamison, D. T., Murray, C. J. Global and regional burden of disease and risk factors, 2001: Systematic analysis of population health data. *Lancet.* 2006;367:1747-1757.

[15] Simmons, B. B., Gadegbeku, A. B., Cirignano, B. Transient ischemic attack: Part ii. Risk factor modification and treatment. *American family physician.* 2012;86:527-532.

[16] De Backer, G., Ambrosioni, E., Borch-Johnsen, K., Brotons, C., Cifkova, R., Dallongeville, J., et al. European guidelines on cardiovascular disease and prevention in clinical practice. *Atherosclerosis.* 2003;171:145-155.

[17] Eckstein, H. H., Kuhnl, A., Dorfler, A., Kopp, I. B., Lawall, H., Ringleb, P. A. The diagnosis, treatment and follow-up of extracranial carotid stenosis: A multidisciplinary german-austrian guideline based on evidence and consensus. *Deutsches Arzteblatt international.* 2013;110: 468-476.

[18] Bonaca, M. P., Beckman, J. Management of asymptomatic carotid artery stenosis. *Current treatment options in cardiovascular medicine.* 2013; 15:252-263.

[19] He, J., Ogden, L. G., Vupputuri, S., Bazzano, L. A., Loria, C., Whelton, P. K. Dietary sodium intake and subsequent risk of cardiovascular disease in overweight adults. *JAMA: the journal of the American Medical Association.* 1999;282:2027-2034.

[20] Constantinou, J., Jayia, P., Hamilton, G. Best evidence for medical therapy for carotid artery stenosis. *Journal of vascular surgery*. 2013;58: 1129-1139.

[21] MacGregor, G. A., Markandu, N. D., Sagnella, G. A., Singer, D. R., Cappuccio, F. P. Double-blind study of three sodium intakes and long-term effects of sodium restriction in essential hypertension. *Lancet*. 1989;2:1244-1247.

[22] Sacks, F. M., Svetkey, L. P., Vollmer, W. M., Appel, L. J., Bray, G. A., Harsha, D., et al. Effects on blood pressure of reduced dietary sodium and the dietary approaches to stop hypertension (dash) diet. Dash-sodium collaborative research group. *The New England journal of medicine*. 2001;344:3-10.

[23] Vollmer, W. M., Sacks, F. M., Ard, J., Appel, L. J., Bray, G. A., Simons-Morton, D. G., et al. Effects of diet and sodium intake on blood pressure: Subgroup analysis of the dash-sodium trial. *Annals of internal medicine*. 2001;135:1019-1028.

[24] Whelton, P. K., He, J., Cutler, J. A., Brancati, F. L., Appel, L. J., Follmann, D., et al. Effects of oral potassium on blood pressure. Meta-analysis of randomized controlled clinical trials. *JAMA: the journal of the American Medical Association*. 1997;277:1624-1632.

[25] Manson, J. E., Colditz, G. A., Stampfer, M. J., Willett, W. C., Krolewski, A. S., Rosner, B., et al. A prospective study of maturity-onset diabetes mellitus and risk of coronary heart disease and stroke in women. *Archives of internal medicine*. 1991;151:1141-1147.

[26] Blair, S. N., Kampert, J. B., Kohl, H. W., 3rd, Barlow, C. E., Macera, C. A., Paffenbarger, R. S., Jr., et al. Influences of cardiorespiratory fitness and other precursors on cardiovascular disease and all-cause mortality in men and women. *JAMA: the journal of the American Medical Association*. 1996;276:205-210.

[27] Endres, M., Gertz, K., Lindauer, U., Katchanov, J., Schultze, J., Schrock, H., et al. Mechanisms of stroke protection by physical activity. *Annals of neurology*. 2003;54:582-590.

[28] Dylewicz, P., Przywarska, I., Szczesniak, L., Rychlewski, T., Bienkowska, S., Dlugiewicz, I., et al. The influence of short-term endurance training on the insulin blood level, binding, and degradation of 125i-insulin by erythrocyte receptors in patients after myocardial infarction. *Journal of cardiopulmonary rehabilitation*. 1999;19:98-105.

[29] Williams, M. A., Fleg, J. L., Ades, P. A., Chaitman, B. R., Miller, N. H., Mohiuddin, S. M., et al. Secondary prevention of coronary heart disease

in the elderly (with emphasis on patients > or =75 years of age): An american heart association scientific statement from the council on clinical cardiology subcommittee on exercise, cardiac rehabilitation, and prevention. *Circulation*. 2002;105:1735-1743.

[30] Lakka, T. A., Salonen, J. T. Moderate to high intensity conditioning leisure time physical activity and high cardiorespiratory fitness are associated with reduced plasma fibrinogen in eastern finnish men. *Journal of clinical epidemiology*. 1993;46:1119-1127.

[31] Wang, H. Y., Bashore, T. R., Friedman, E. Exercise reduces age-dependent decrease in platelet protein kinase c activity and translocation. *The journals of gerontology. Series A, Biological sciences and medical sciences*. 1995;50A:M12-16.

[32] Williams, P. T. High-density lipoprotein cholesterol and other risk factors for coronary heart disease in female runners. *The New England journal of medicine*. 1996;334:1298-1303.

[33] Lee, C. D., Folsom, A. R., Blair, S. N. Physical activity and stroke risk: A meta-analysis. *Stroke; a journal of cerebral circulation*. 2003;34: 2475-2481.

[34] Thompson, P. D., Buchner, D., Pina, I. L., Balady, G. J., Williams, M. A., Marcus, B. H., et al. Exercise and physical activity in the prevention and treatment of atherosclerotic cardiovascular disease: A statement from the council on clinical cardiology (subcommittee on exercise, rehabilitation, and prevention) and the council on nutrition, physical activity, and metabolism (subcommittee on physical activity). *Circulation*. 2003;107:3109-3116.

[35] Brott, T. G., Halperin, J. L., Abbara, S., Bacharach, J. M., Barr, J. D., Bush, R. L., et al. 2011 asa/accf/aha/aann/aans/acr/asnr/cns/saip/scai/sir/ snis/svm/svs guideline on the management of patients with extracranial carotid and vertebral artery disease: A report of the american college of cardiology foundation/american heart association task force on practice guidelines, and the american stroke association, american association of neuroscience nurses, american association of neurological surgeons, american college of radiology, american society of neuroradiology, congress of neurological surgeons, society of atherosclerosis imaging and prevention, society for cardiovascular angiography and interventions, society of interventional radiology, society of neurointerventional surgery, society for vascular medicine, and society for vascular surgery. *Journal of the American College of Cardiology*. 2011;57:e16-94.

[36] Sacco, R. L., Gan, R., Boden-Albala, B., Lin, I. F., Kargman, D. E., Hauser, W. A., et al. Leisure-time physical activity and ischemic stroke risk: The northern manhattan stroke study. *Stroke; a journal of cerebral circulation*. 1998;29:380-387.

[37] Tanaka, H., Seals, D. R., Monahan, K. D., Clevenger, C. M., DeSouza, C. A., Dinenno, F. A. Regular aerobic exercise and the age-related increase in carotid artery intima-media thickness in healthy men. *Journal of applied physiology*. 2002;92:1458-1464.

[38] Lakka, T. A., Laukkanen, J. A., Rauramaa, R., Salonen, R., Lakka, H. M., Kaplan, G. A., et al. Cardiorespiratory fitness and the progression of carotid atherosclerosis in middle-aged men. *Annals of internal medicine*. 2001;134:12-20.

[39] Kronenberg, F., Pereira, M. A., Schmitz, M. K., Arnett, D. K., Evenson, K. R., Crapo, R. O., et al. Influence of leisure time physical activity and television watching on atherosclerosis risk factors in the nhlbi family heart study. *Atherosclerosis*. 2000;153:433-443.

[40] Fine-Edelstein, J. S., Wolf, P. A., O'Leary, D. H., Poehlman, H., Belanger, A. J., Kase, C. S., et al. Precursors of extracranial carotid atherosclerosis in the framingham study. *Neurology*. 1994;44:1046-1050.

[41] Dobs, A. S., Nieto, F. J., Szklo, M., Barnes, R., Sharrett, A. R., Ko, W. J. Risk factors for popliteal and carotid wall thicknesses in the atherosclerosis risk in communities (aric) study. *American journal of epidemiology*. 1999;150:1055-1067.

[42] O'Leary, D. H., Polak, J. F., Kronmal, R. A., Savage, P. J., Borhani, N. O., Kittner, S. J., et al. Thickening of the carotid wall. A marker for atherosclerosis in the elderly? Cardiovascular health study collaborative research group. *Stroke; a journal of cerebral circulation*. 1996;27:224-231.

[43] Djousse, L., Myers, R. H., Province, M. A., Hunt, S. C., Eckfeldt, J. H., Evans, G., et al. Influence of apolipoprotein e, smoking, and alcohol intake on carotid atherosclerosis: National heart, lung, and blood institute family heart study. *Stroke; a journal of cerebral circulation*. 2002;33:1357-1361.

[44] Howard, G., Wagenknecht, L. E., Cai, J., Cooper, L., Kraut, M. A., Toole, J. F. Cigarette smoking and other risk factors for silent cerebral infarction in the general population. *Stroke; a journal of cerebral circulation*. 1998;29:913-917.

[45] Wilson, P. W., Hoeg, J. M., D'Agostino, R. B., Silbershatz, H., Belanger, A. M., Poehlmann, H., et al. Cumulative effects of high cholesterol levels, high blood pressure, and cigarette smoking on carotid stenosis. *The New England journal of medicine.* 1997;337:516-522.

[46] Tell, G. S., Rutan, G. H., Kronmal, R. A., Bild, D. E., Polak, J. F., Wong, N. D., et al. Correlates of blood pressure in community-dwelling older adults. The cardiovascular health study. Cardiovascular health study (chs) collaborative research group. *Hypertension.* 1994;23:59-67.

[47] Ritter, J. C., Tyrrell, M. R. The current management of carotid atherosclerotic disease: Who, when and how? *Interactive cardiovascular and thoracic surgery.* 2013;16:339-346.

[48] Winter, Y., Rohrmann, S., Linseisen, J., Lanczik, O., Ringleb, P. A., Hebebrand, J., et al. Contribution of obesity and abdominal fat mass to risk of stroke and transient ischemic attacks. *Stroke; a journal of cerebral circulation.* 2008;39:3145-3151.

[49] Expert Panel on Detection E, Treatment of High Blood Cholesterol in A. Executive summary of the third report of the national cholesterol education program (ncep) expert panel on detection, evaluation, and treatment of high blood cholesterol in adults (adult treatment panel iii). *JAMA: the journal of the American Medical Association.* 2001;285: 2486-2497.

[50] McNeill, A. M., Rosamond, W. D., Girman, C. J., Heiss, G., Golden, S. H., Duncan, B. B., et al. Prevalence of coronary heart disease and carotid arterial thickening in patients with the metabolic syndrome (the aric study). *The American journal of cardiology.* 2004;94:1249-1254.

[51] Kawamoto, R., Ohtsuka, N., Ninomiya, D., Nakamura, S. Carotid atherosclerosis in normal-weight metabolic syndrome. *Internal medicine.* 2007;46:1771-1777.

[52] Scuteri, A., Najjar, S. S., Muller, D. C., Andres, R., Hougaku, H., Metter, E. J., et al. Metabolic syndrome amplifies the age-associated increases in vascular thickness and stiffness. *Journal of the American College of Cardiology.* 2004;43:1388-1395.

[53] Kawamoto, R., Tomita, H., Oka, Y., Kodama, A., Kamitani, A. Metabolic syndrome amplifies the ldl-cholesterol associated increases in carotid atherosclerosis. *Internal medicine.* 2005;44:1232-1238.

[54] Kawamoto, R., Tomita, H., Oka, Y., Ohtsuka, N., Kamitani, A. Metabolic syndrome and carotid atherosclerosis: Role of elevated blood pressure. *Journal of atherosclerosis and thrombosis.* 2005;12:268-275.

[55] Irace, C., Cortese, C., Fiaschi, E., Carallo, C., Sesti, G., Farinaro, E., et al. Components of the metabolic syndrome and carotid atherosclerosis: Role of elevated blood pressure. *Hypertension.* 2005;45:597-601.

[56] Teramura, M., Emoto, M., Araki, T., Yokoyama, H., Motoyama, K., Shinohara, K., et al. Clinical impact of metabolic syndrome by modified ncep-atpiii criteria on carotid atherosclerosis in japanese adults. *Journal of atherosclerosis and thrombosis.* 2007;14:172-178.

[57] Empana, J. P., Zureik, M., Gariepy, J., Courbon, D., Dartigues, J. F., Ritchie, K., et al. The metabolic syndrome and the carotid artery structure in noninstitutionalized elderly subjects: The three-city study. *Stroke; a journal of cerebral circulation.* 2007;38:893-899.

[58] Smith, N. L., Barzilay, J. I., Shaffer, D., Savage, P. J., Heckbert, S. R., Kuller, L. H., et al. Fasting and 2-hour postchallenge serum glucose measures and risk of incident cardiovascular events in the elderly: The cardiovascular health study. *Archives of internal medicine.* 2002;162: 209-216.

[59] O'Leary, D. H., Polak, J. F., Kronmal, R. A., Kittner, S. J., Bond, M. G., Wolfson, S. K., Jr., et al. Distribution and correlates of sonographically detected carotid artery disease in the cardiovascular health study. The chs collaborative research group. *Stroke; a journal of cerebral circulation.* 1992;23:1752-1760.

[60] Wagenknecht, L. E., D'Agostino, R., Jr., Savage, P. J., O'Leary, D. H., Saad, M. F., Haffner, S. M. Duration of diabetes and carotid wall thickness. The insulin resistance atherosclerosis study (iras). *Stroke; a journal of cerebral circulation.* 1997;28:999-1005.

[61] Haffner, S. M., Agostino, R. D., Jr., Saad, M. F., O'Leary, D. H., Savage, P. J., Rewers, M., et al. Carotid artery atherosclerosis in type-2 diabetic and nondiabetic subjects with and without symptomatic coronary artery disease (the insulin resistance atherosclerosis study). *The American journal of cardiology.* 2000;85:1395-1400.

[62] Folsom, A. R., Rasmussen, M. L., Chambless, L. E., Howard, G., Cooper, L. S., Schmidt, M. I., et al. Prospective associations of fasting insulin, body fat distribution, and diabetes with risk of ischemic stroke. The atherosclerosis risk in communities (aric) study investigators. *Diabetes care.* 1999;22:1077-1083.

[63] Chambless, L. E., Folsom, A. R., Davis, V., Sharrett, R., Heiss, G., Sorlie, P., et al. Risk factors for progression of common carotid atherosclerosis: The atherosclerosis risk in communities study, 1987-1998. *American journal of epidemiology.* 2002;155:38-47.

[64] Langenfeld, M. R., Forst, T., Hohberg, C., Kann, P., Lubben, G., Konrad, T., et al. Pioglitazone decreases carotid intima-media thickness independently of glycemic control in patients with type 2 diabetes mellitus: Results from a controlled randomized study. *Circulation*. 2005; 111:2525-2531.

[65] Mazzone, T., Meyer, P. M., Feinstein, S. B., Davidson, M. H., Kondos, G. T., D'Agostino, R. B., Sr., et al. Effect of pioglitazone compared with glimepiride on carotid intima-media thickness in type 2 diabetes: A randomized trial. *JAMA: the journal of the American Medical Association*. 2006;296:2572-2581.

[66] Nathan, D. M., Lachin, J., Cleary, P., Orchard, T., Brillon, D. J., Backlund, J. Y., et al. Intensive diabetes therapy and carotid intima-media thickness in type 1 diabetes mellitus. *The New England journal of medicine*. 2003;348:2294-2303.

[67] Skyler, J. S., Bergenstal, R., Bonow, R. O., Buse, J., Deedwania, P., Gale, E. A., et al. Intensive glycemic control and the prevention of cardiovascular events: Implications of the accord, advance, and va diabetes trials: A position statement of the american diabetes association and a scientific statement of the american college of cardiology foundation and the american heart association. *Journal of the American College of Cardiology*. 2009;53:298-304.

[68] Kelly, T. N., Bazzano, L. A., Fonseca, V. A., Thethi, T. K., Reynolds, K., He, J. Systematic review: Glucose control and cardiovascular disease in type 2 diabetes. *Annals of internal medicine*. 2009;151:394-403.

[69] Kernan, W. N., Inzucchi, S. E. Type 2 diabetes mellitus and insulin resistance: Stroke prevention and management. *Current treatment options in neurology*. 2004;6:443-450.

[70] James, P. A., Oparil, S., Carter, B. L., Cushman, W. C., Dennison-Himmelfarb, C., Handler, J., et al. 2014 evidence-based guideline for the management of high blood pressure in adults: Report from the panel members appointed to the eighth joint national committee (jnc 8). *JAMA: the journal of the American Medical Association*. 2014;311:507-520.

[71] Endres, M., Heuschmann, P. U., Laufs, U., Hakim, A. M. Primary prevention of stroke: Blood pressure, lipids, and heart failure. *European heart journal*. 2011;32:545-552.

[72] Lawes, C. M., Bennett, D. A., Feigin, V. L., Rodgers, A. Blood pressure and stroke: An overview of published reviews. *Stroke; a journal of cerebral circulation*. 2004;35:1024.

[73] Rashid, P., Leonardi-Bee, J., Bath, P. Blood pressure reduction and secondary prevention of stroke and other vascular events: A systematic review. *Stroke; a journal of cerebral circulation.* 2003;34:2741-2748.

[74] Yusuf, S., Sleight, P., Pogue, J., Bosch, J., Davies, R., Dagenais, G. Effects of an angiotensin-converting-enzyme inhibitor, ramipril, on cardiovascular events in high-risk patients. The heart outcomes prevention evaluation study investigators. *The New England journal of medicine.* 2000;342:145-153.

[75] Heiss, G., Sharrett, A. R., Barnes, R., Chambless, L. E., Szklo, M., Alzola, C. Carotid atherosclerosis measured by b-mode ultrasound in populations: Associations with cardiovascular risk factors in the aric study. *American journal of epidemiology.* 1991;134:250-256.

[76] Sacco, R. L., Roberts, J. K., Boden-Albala, B., Gu, Q., Lin, I. F., Kargman, D. E., et al. Race-ethnicity and determinants of carotid atherosclerosis in a multiethnic population. The northern manhattan stroke study. *Stroke; a journal of cerebral circulation.* 1997;28:929-935.

[77] Sharrett, A. R., Patsch, W., Sorlie, P. D., Heiss, G., Bond, M. G., Davis, C. E. Associations of lipoprotein cholesterols, apolipoproteins a-i and b, and triglycerides with carotid atherosclerosis and coronary heart disease. The atherosclerosis risk in communities (aric) study. *Arteriosclerosis and thrombosis: a journal of vascular biology / American Heart Association.* 1994;14:1098-1104.

[78] Davies, K. N., Humphrey, P. R. Complications of cerebral angiography in patients with symptomatic carotid territory ischaemia screened by carotid ultrasound. *Journal of neurology, neurosurgery, and psychiatry.* 1993;56:967-972.

[79] Endres, M. Statins and stroke. *Journal of cerebral blood flow and metabolism: official journal of the International Society of Cerebral Blood Flow and Metabolism.* 2005;25:1093-1110.

[80] Amarenco, P., Labreuche, J., Lavallee, P., Touboul, P. J. Statins in stroke prevention and carotid atherosclerosis: Systematic review and up-to-date meta-analysis. *Stroke; a journal of cerebral circulation.* 2004;35: 2902-2909.

[81] Crouse, J. R., 3rd, Raichlen, J. S., Riley, W. A., Evans, G. W., Palmer, M. K., O'Leary, D. H., et al. Effect of rosuvastatin on progression of carotid intima-media thickness in low-risk individuals with subclinical atherosclerosis: The meteor trial. *JAMA: the journal of the American Medical Association.* 2007;297:1344-1353.

[82] Smilde, T. J., van Wissen, S., Wollersheim, H., Trip, M. D., Kastelein, J. J., Stalenhoef, A. F. Effect of aggressive versus conventional lipid lowering on atherosclerosis progression in familial hypercholesterolaemia (asap): A prospective, randomised, double-blind trial. *Lancet.* 2001;357:577-581.

[83] Taylor, A. J., Kent, S. M., Flaherty, P. J., Coyle, L. C., Markwood, T. T., Vernalis, M. N. Arbiter: Arterial biology for the investigation of the treatment effects of reducing cholesterol: A randomized trial comparing the effects of atorvastatin and pravastatin on carotid intima medial thickness. *Circulation.* 2002;106:2055-2060.

[84] Amarenco, P., Bogousslavsky, J., Callahan, A., 3rd, Goldstein, L. B., Hennerici, M., Rudolph, A. E., et al. High-dose atorvastatin after stroke or transient ischemic attack. *The New England journal of medicine.* 2006;355:549-559.

[85] Sillesen, H., Amarenco, P., Hennerici, M. G., Callahan, A., Goldstein, L. B., Zivin, J., et al. Atorvastatin reduces the risk of cardiovascular events in patients with carotid atherosclerosis: A secondary analysis of the stroke prevention by aggressive reduction in cholesterol levels (sparcl) trial. *Stroke; a journal of cerebral circulation.* 2008;39:3297-3302.

[86] Heart Protection Study Collaborative G. Mrc/bhf heart protection study of cholesterol lowering with simvastatin in 20,536 high-risk individuals: A randomised placebo-controlled trial. *Lancet.* 2002;360:7-22.

[87] Blankenhorn, D. H., Selzer, R. H., Crawford, D. W., Barth, J. D., Liu, C. R., Liu, C. H., et al. Beneficial effects of colestipol-niacin therapy on the common carotid artery. Two- and four-year reduction of intima-media thickness measured by ultrasound. *Circulation.* 1993;88:20-28.

[88] Taylor, A. J., Sullenberger, L. E., Lee, H. J., Lee, J. K., Grace, K. A. Arterial biology for the investigation of the treatment effects of reducing cholesterol (arbiter) 2: A double-blind, placebo-controlled study of extended-release niacin on atherosclerosis progression in secondary prevention patients treated with statins. *Circulation.* 2004;110:3512-3517.

[89] Antithrombotic Trialists C. Collaborative meta-analysis of randomised trials of antiplatelet therapy for prevention of death, myocardial infarction, and stroke in high risk patients. *Bmj.* 2002;324:71-86.

[90] Sandercock, P. A., Counsell, C., Kamal, A. K. Anticoagulants for acute ischaemic stroke. *The Cochrane database of systematic reviews.* 2008: CD000024.

[91] Hobson, R. W., 2nd, Weiss, D. G., Fields, W. S., Goldstone, J., Moore, W. S., Towne, J. B., et al. Efficacy of carotid endarterectomy for asymptomatic carotid stenosis. The veterans affairs cooperative study group. *The New England journal of medicine.* 1993;328:221-227.

[92] Endarterectomy for asymptomatic carotid artery stenosis. Executive committee for the asymptomatic carotid atherosclerosis study. *JAMA: the journal of the American Medical Association.* 1995;273:1421-1428.

[93] Goldstein, L. B., Adams, R., Becker, K., Furberg, C. D., Gorelick, P. B., Hademenos, G., et al. Primary prevention of ischemic stroke: A statement for healthcare professionals from the stroke council of the american heart association. *Stroke; a journal of cerebral circulation.* 2001;32:280-299.

[94] Campbell, C. L., Smyth, S., Montalescot, G., Steinhubl, S. R. Aspirin dose for the prevention of cardiovascular disease: A systematic review. *JAMA: the journal of the American Medical Association.* 2007;297: 2018-2024.

[95] Antithrombotic Trialists, C., Baigent, C., Blackwell, L., Collins, R., Emberson, J., Godwin, J., et al. Aspirin in the primary and secondary prevention of vascular disease: Collaborative meta-analysis of individual participant data from randomised trials. *Lancet.* 2009;373:1849-1860.

[96] Halkes, P. H., Gray, L. J., Bath, P. M., Diener, H. C., Guiraud-Chaumeil, B., Yatsu, F. M., et al. Dipyridamole plus aspirin versus aspirin alone in secondary prevention after tia or stroke: A meta-analysis by risk. *Journal of neurology, neurosurgery, and psychiatry.* 2008;79:1218-1223.

[97] Thijs, V., Lemmens, R., Fieuws, S. Network meta-analysis: Simultaneous meta-analysis of common antiplatelet regimens after transient ischaemic attack or stroke. *European heart journal.* 2008;29: 1086-1092.

[98] Chan, F. K., Ching, J. Y., Hung, L. C., Wong, V. W., Leung, V. K., Kung, N. N., et al. Clopidogrel versus aspirin and esomeprazole to prevent recurrent ulcer bleeding. *The New England journal of medicine.* 2005;352:238-244.

[99] Sacco, R. L., Adams, R., Albers, G., Alberts, M. J., Benavente, O., Furie, K., et al. Guidelines for prevention of stroke in patients with ischemic stroke or transient ischemic attack. A statement for healthcare professionals from the american heart association/american stroke association council on stroke: Co-sponsored by the council on cardiovascular radiology and intervention: The american academy of

neurology affirms the value of this guideline. *Circulation.* 2006;113: e409-449.

[100] North American Symptomatic Carotid Endarterectomy Trial C. Beneficial effect of carotid endarterectomy in symptomatic patients with high-grade carotid stenosis. *The New England journal of medicine.* 1991;325:445-453.

[101] Bhatt, D. L., Fox, K. A., Hacke, W., Berger, P. B., Black, H. R., Boden, W. E., et al. Clopidogrel and aspirin versus aspirin alone for the prevention of atherothrombotic events. *The New England journal of medicine.* 2006;354:1706-1717.

[102] Diener, H. C., Bogousslavsky, J., Brass, L. M., Cimminiello, C., Csiba, L., Kaste, M., et al. Aspirin and clopidogrel compared with clopidogrel alone after recent ischaemic stroke or transient ischaemic attack in high-risk patients (match): Randomised, double-blind, placebo-controlled trial. *Lancet.* 2004;364:331-337.

[103] Investigators, S. P. S., Benavente, O. R., Hart, R. G., McClure, L. A., Szychowski, J. M., Coffey, C. S., et al. Effects of clopidogrel added to aspirin in patients with recent lacunar stroke. *The New England journal of medicine.* 2012;367:817-825.

[104] Dinicolantonio, J. J., Lavie, C. J., Fares, H., Menezes, A. R., O'Keefe, J. H., Bangalore, S., et al. Meta-analysis of cilostazol versus aspirin for the secondary prevention of stroke. *The American journal of cardiology.* 2013;112:1230-1234.

[105] Yamagami, H., Sakai, N., Matsumaru, Y., Sakai, C., Kai, Y., Sugiu, K., et al. Periprocedural cilostazol treatment and restenosis after carotid artery stenting: The retrospective study of in-stent restenosis after carotid artery stenting (resister-cas). *Journal of stroke and cerebrovascular diseases: the official journal of National Stroke Association.* 2012;21:193-199.

[106] De Schryver, E. L., Algra, A., Kappelle, L. J., van Gijn, J., Koudstaal, P. J. Vitamin k antagonists versus antiplatelet therapy after transient ischaemic attack or minor ischaemic stroke of presumed arterial origin. *The Cochrane database of systematic reviews.* 2012;9:CD001342.

[107] Mohr, J. P., Thompson, J. L., Lazar, R. M., Levin, B., Sacco, R. L., Furie, K. L., et al. A comparison of warfarin and aspirin for the prevention of recurrent ischemic stroke. *The New England journal of medicine.* 2001;345:1444-1451.

[108] Ntaios, G. C., Savopoulos, C. G., Chatzinikolaou, A. C., Kaiafa, G. D., Hatzitolios, A. Vitamins and stroke: The homocysteine hypothesis still in doubt. *The neurologist.* 2008;14:2-4.

[109] Ntaios, G., Savopoulos, C., Grekas, D., Hatzitolios, A. The controversial role of b-vitamins in cardiovascular risk: An update. *Archives of cardiovascular diseases.* 2009;102:847-854.

[110] Ntaios, G., Savopoulos, C., Chatzopoulos, S., Mikhailidis, D., Hatzitolios, A. Iatrogenic hyperhomocysteinemia in patients with metabolic syndrome: A systematic review and metaanalysis. *Atherosclerosis.* 2011;214:11-19.

[111] Malinow, M. R., Nieto, F. J., Szklo, M., Chambless, L. E., Bond, G. Carotid artery intimal-medial wall thickening and plasma homocyst(e)ine in asymptomatic adults. The atherosclerosis risk in communities study. *Circulation.* 1993;87:1107-1113.

[112] Potter, K., Hankey, G. J., Green, D. J., Eikelboom, J., Jamrozik, K., Arnolda, L. F. The effect of long-term homocysteine-lowering on carotid intima-media thickness and flow-mediated vasodilation in stroke patients: A randomized controlled trial and meta-analysis. *BMC cardiovascular disorders.* 2008;8:24

[113] Ntaios, G., Chatzinikolaou, A., Savopoulos, C., Hatzitolios, A. "Well done folate, the little boy was born healthy without spina bifida: But will he suffer a stroke when elderly?". *European journal of internal medicine.* 2009;20:2.

[114] Ntaios, G., Savopoulos, C., Hatzitolios, A., Chatzinikolaou, A., Karamitsos, D. Is there a beneficial effect of folic acid on carotid intima-media thickness? *International journal of cardiology.* 2009;135:260-261.

[115] Ntaios, G., Savopoulos, C., Karamitsos, D., Economou, I., Destanis, E., Chryssogonidis, I., et al. The effect of folic acid supplementation on carotid intima-media thickness in patients with cardiovascular risk: A randomized, placebo-controlled trial. *International journal of cardiology.* 2010;143.16-19.

[116] Hodis, H. N., Mack, W. J., Dustin, L., Mahrer, P. R., Azen, S. P., Detrano, R., et al. High-dose b vitamin supplementation and progression of subclinical atherosclerosis: A randomized controlled trial. *Stroke; a journal of cerebral circulation.* 2009;40.730-736.

[117] Zoungas, S., McGrath, B. P., Branley, P., Kerr, P. G., Muske, C., Wolfe, R., et al. Cardiovascular morbidity and mortality in the atherosclerosis and folic acid supplementation trial (asfast) in chronic renal failure: A

multicenter, randomized, controlled trial. *Journal of the American College of Cardiology*. 2006;47:1108-1116.

[118] Ariyo, A. A., Thach, C., Tracy, R., Cardiovascular Health Study I. Lp(a) lipoprotein, vascular disease, and mortality in the elderly. *The New England journal of medicine*. 2003;349:2108-2115.

[119] Willeit, J., Kiechl, S., Santer, P., Oberhollenzer, F., Egger, G., Jarosch, E., et al. Lipoprotein(a) and asymptomatic carotid artery disease. Evidence of a prominent role in the evolution of advanced carotid plaques: The bruneck study. *Stroke; a journal of cerebral circulation*. 1995;26:1582-1587.

[120] Ridker, P. M., Cushman, M., Stampfer, M. J., Tracy, R. P., Hennekens, C. H. Inflammation, aspirin, and the risk of cardiovascular disease in apparently healthy men. *The New England journal of medicine*. 1997; 336:973-979.

[121] Salmon, J. E., Roman, M. J. Subclinical atherosclerosis in rheumatoid arthritis and systemic lupus erythematosus. *The American journal of medicine*. 2008;121:S3-8.

[122] Roman, M. J., Moeller, E., Davis, A., Paget, S. A., Crow, M. K., Lockshin, M. D., et al. Preclinical carotid atherosclerosis in patients with rheumatoid arthritis. *Annals of internal medicine*. 2006;144:249-256.

[123] Manzi, S., Selzer, F., Sutton-Tyrrell, K., Fitzgerald, S. G., Rairie, J. E., Tracy, R. P., et al. Prevalence and risk factors of carotid plaque in women with systemic lupus erythematosus. *Arthritis and rheumatism*. 1999;42:51-60.

[124] Inzitari, D., Eliasziw, M., Gates, P., Sharpe, B. L., Chan, R. K., Meldrum, H. E., et al. The causes and risk of stroke in patients with asymptomatic internal-carotid-artery stenosis. North american symptomatic carotid endarterectomy trial collaborators. *The New England journal of medicine*. 2000;342:1693-1700.

[125] Halliday, A., Harrison, M., Hayter, E., Kong, X., Mansfield, A., Marro, J., et al. 10-year stroke prevention after successful carotid endarterectomy for asymptomatic stenosis (acst-1): A multicentre randomised trial. *Lancet*. 2010;376:1074-1084.

In: Carotid Artery Disease   ISBN: 978-1-63321-859-8
Editor: Sherri Derricks   © 2014 Nova Science Publishers, Inc.

Chapter 2

Intracranial Carotid Artery Stenosis Diagnosed with CTA in a Western Population: Predictor for Poor Outcome

Wessel E. van der Steen, MSc[1,*],
Jan-Dirk Vermeij, MD[1,†], *Henk A. Marquering, PhD*[2,††],
René van den Berg, PhD, MD[3,‡],
Charles B. Majoie, PhD, MD[3,#] *and*
Paul J. Nederkoorn, PhD, MD[1,•]

[1]Department of Neurology, Academic Medical
Center (AMC), Amsterdam, the Netherlands
[2]Department of Biomedical Engineering and Physics
and department of Radiology, Academic Medical
Center (AMC), Amsterdam, the Netherlands
[3]Department of Radiology, Academic Medical Center (AMC),
Amsterdam, the Netherlands

* Wessel E. van der Steen, MSc. E-mail: w.e.vandersteen@amc.uva.nl.
† Jan-Dirk Vermeij, MD. E-mail: j.d.vermeij@amc.uva.nl.
†† Henk A. Marquering, PhD. E-mail: h.a.marquering@amc.uva.nl.
‡ René van den Berg, PhD, MD. E-mail: r.vdberg@amc.uva.nl.
# Charles B. Majoie, PhD, MD. E-mail: c.b.majoie@amc.uva.nl.
• Paul J. Nederkoorn, PhD, MD. E-mail: p.j.nederkoorn@amc.uva.nl.

Abstract

Background: The prevalence and impact of intracranial atherosclerosis in the white population is sparsely researched and optimal treatment remains to be defined. Previously, we found that 84% of the patients with extracranial internal carotid artery (ICA) stenosis also had an intracranial ICA stenosis diagnosed with CT angiography (CTA).

The purpose of this chapter is to investigate the relation between intracranial ICA stenosis and outcome.

Methods: We conducted a single center cohort study with long-term follow-up of 84 patients with TIA or infarct that underwent a CTA for the assessment of a carotid artery stenosis between April 1, 2006 and December 31, 2008. Intracranial ICA stenosis was categorised in four groups: without any stenosis (<30%), with any stenosis ($\geq$ 30%), without severe stenosis (<70%), and with severe stenosis ($\geq$ 70%), Primary outcome was recurrent TIA or infarct. Secondary outcomes were MI, vascular death and functional outcome. Poor functional outcome was defined as mRS $\geq$3.

Results: Mean follow-up in the 84 patients was 4.1 years ($\pm$1.2 years). Comparing patients without stenosis to patients with any stenosis ($\geq$30%), no differences in primary and secondary outcomes were found. Severe stenosis ($\geq$70%) was not associated with recurrent stroke, but was strongly associated with vascular death (OR 7.85 (1.9 - 32.5)) and poor functional outcome (OR 4.33 (1.15 - 16.37)).

Conclusion: Severe intracranial ICA stenosis on CTA in a white population is associated with a higher rate of vascular death and poor functional outcome.

Introduction

The presence of atherosclerotic disease in the extracranial part of the internal carotid artery (ICA) is a strong predictor for recurrent ischemic stroke in patients who have recently had symptoms (TIA or stroke). [1] It has been shown that the presence of intracranial atherosclerosis also is an independent risk factor for recurrent stroke, especially in blacks, Asians and Hispanics. [2] However, the prevalence and prognosis of intracranial atherosclerosis in the western (mainly white) population is still sparsely studied and optimal treatment remains to be defined. [3]

Kappelle et al. reported intracranial atherosclerosis in one third of the patients with symptomatic extracranial stenosis. [4]

Wityk et al. found a prevalence of intracranial stenosis of 24%. [5]

The diagnosis of an intracranial stenosis in these studies was based on evaluation with Digital Subtraction Angiography (DSA) and Transcranial Doppler (TCD). CT angiography (CTA) allows the assessment of the full 3D morphology of the intracranial vasculature. [6-8] Few studies determined the prevalence of intracranial stenosis using CTA. Recently, we reported a much higher prevalence of intracranial ICA stenosis on 64-section CTA compared with earlier publications: 84% for a degree of stenosis of ≥30% and 39% for a degree of stenosis of ≥50%. [4, 5, 9]

The clinical relevance of the presence of intracranial ICA stenosis on CTA images remains to be elucidated, the purpose of this chapter is to determine the relation between the presence of intracranial ICA stenosis on CTA images and the rate of recurrent stroke and other neurological, cardiovascular and functional outcomes.

Materials and Methods

Study Design

We conducted a single center cohort study with long-term follow-up of all consecutive patients with TIA or infarct that underwent a CT angiography on a 64-section CT scanner for the assessment of a carotid artery stenosis between April 1, 2006 and December 31, 2008.

Study Population

According to our current hospital guidelines, a duplex ultrasound examination was performed in all patients with a TIA or a cerebral infarct, suspected of having a carotid artery stenosis. If this duplex showed an extracranial stenosis of ≥30% in men and ≥50% in women, subsequent CTA was performed. [10] All consecutive patients that underwent a CTA on a 64-section CT scanner (Brilliance 64, Philips Healthcare, Best, the Netherlands) in the Academic Medical Center (AMC) under suspicion of a symptomatic carotid artery stenosis between April 2006 and December 2008 were included in our study. Patients were excluded if there was a history of previous carotid endarterectomy or stenting, and if the images of the CTA studies were of insufficient quality. [9]

CTA Analysis

The degree of intracranial carotid artery stenosis was measured by an experienced neuroradiologist according to the Warfarin-Aspirin Symptomatic Intracranial Disease (WASID) criteria. [10] The most severe intracranial ICA narrowing of both carotid arteries was used as measurement for degree of intracranial ICA stenosis. For the comparative analyses four groups were defined: without any stenosis ($< 30\%$), with any stenosis ($\geq 30\%$), without severe stenosis ($< 70\%$), and with severe stenosis ($\geq 70\%$).

Baseline Characteristics

Baseline characteristics included age, sex, ethnicity, index event (TIA, cerebral infarct or amaurosis fugax), cardiovascular risk profile (blood pressure, diabetes, smoking habit, and cholesterol), carotid interventions after the index event, and a history of cerebrovascular-, cardiovascular- and peripheral vascular disease. [11] Hypertension was defined as a clinical history of systolic blood pressure ≥ 140 mm Hg or diastolic blood pressure ≥ 90 mm Hg or the use of blood pressure lowering medication.

Diabetes was defined as a serum glucose level of ≥ 7.9 mmol/L or treatment with antidiabetic medication. Hypercholesterolemia was defined as a clinical history of hypercholesterolemia, the use of cholesterol lowering medication or a total cholesterol of ≥ 5.0 mmol/L if no further information could be found. Data was obtained retrospectively from medical records and discharge letters from our hospital.

Outcomes

The primary outcome was rate of recurrent TIA or infarct. If new focal neurological symptoms occurred and resolved within 24 hours without the presence of hemorrhage on radiological imaging of the brain, the event was classified as TIA. If the symptoms lasted longer than 24 hours and imaging showed no abnormalities or an infarct, it was defined as recurrent infarct.

Secondary outcomes were myocardial infarction, vascular death and a combined endpoint (TIA or cerebral infarct, myocardial infarction, and vascular death). Myocardial infarction was defined as symptoms of cardiac ischemia with the rise of cardiac biomarkers.

Vascular death was defined as sudden death or death within 30 days after any of these events: myocardial infarction, pulmonary embolism, rupture of an aortic aneurysm or terminal heart failure. In addition, we assessed the functional outcome, as defined on the modified Rankin Scale (mRS). A mRS-score $\geq$ 3 was considered a poor functional outcome.

Follow-Up

Outcomes were assessed by a structured telephone-interview by a single observer (W.E.S), blinded for all radiological test results. Patients were asked if any recurrent event had occurred. As part of the structured interview, the mRS was assessed. [12, 13] Medical records in our hospital were reviewed to verify if new events reported by the patient met our definitions. The general practitioner was contacted any case of uncertainty, if the patient had died, or if a recurrent event was evaluated in another hospital; the general practitioner was then asked for the discharge letter and additional information.

Statistical Analysis

Baseline differences between patients without any stenosis (<30%) and with any stenosis ($\geq$ 30%) and between patients without severe stenosis (<70%) and with severe stenosis ($\geq$ 70%) were compared using the χ^2 test. We compared the outcomes between the groups without any stenosis (<30%), with any stenosis ($\geq$30%), without severe stenosis (<70%), and with severe stenosis ($\geq$70%), using odds ratio's with 95% confidence interval. Kaplan-Meier survival analysis was used to assess the vascular mortality rate. Kaplan-Meier curves were compared using the Log-Rank test.

All analyses were performed using SPSS Statistics 19.0. A P-value of less than 0.05 was considered statistically significant.

Results

Baseline Characteristics

Eighty-four consecutive patients were included. Baseline characteristics are shown in table 1. Mean age was 67.6 ± 12.6 years and 50 patients (60%) were male. Seventy-six patients (90.4%) were white. There were seven (8%) patients without any stenosis, 77 (92%) with any stenosis, 73 (87%) patients without severe stenosis and 11 (13%) patients with severe stenosis. Regarding the baseline characteristics no significant differences between patients without stenosis and patients with any stenosis were found. Patients with a severe stenosis (≥70%) were significantly more often male, non-white, had a history of coronary artery disease, diabetes and hypercholesteroleamia as compared with patients without a severe stenosis (<70%).

Primary Outcomes

Mean follow-up time was 4.1 (± 1.2) years. A total of 7 recurrent TIA's occurred during the follow-up period. One patient (14%) without any stenosis (<30%) had a recurrent TIA, compared with 6 patients (8%) with any stenosis (≥30%) (OR 0.51 (0.05 - 4.93)). Six recurrent TIA's (8%) occurred in patients without severe stenosis (<70%), compared with 1 (9%) in a patient with severe stenosis (≥70%) (OR 1.12 (0.12 - 10.27)). A total of 11 recurrent infarcts occurred during the follow-up period. All infarcts (14%) occurred in patients with any stenosis (≥30%) (OR 2.59 (0.14 - 48.6)). Ten infarcts (14%) occurred in patients without severe stenosis (<70%), as compared with 1 (9%) in a patient with a severe stenosis (≥70%) (OR 0.63 (0.07 - 5.5)). Table 2 and figure 1 and 2 show the outcomes for the different intracranial ICA stenosis groups.

Secondary Outcomes

Ten patients had a myocardial infarction during the follow-up period. No differences in the occurrence of myocardial infarctions were found comparing patients without any stenosis with patients with any stenosis, and patients with or without a severe stenosis. Fifteen patients deceased during follow-up (18%).

Table 1. Baseline characteristics for patients with and without intracranial ICA stenosis and for patients with and without severe intracranial ICA stenosis

Baseline characteristics	Intracranial internal carotid artery stenosis						
	Total	<30%	≥ 30%	p	<70%	≥ 70%	p
Patient Characteristic	n = 84	n = 7	n = 77		n = 73	n = 11	
Mean Age	67.6 (±12.6)	64.6 (±15.0)	67.9 (±12.5)		67,6 (±12.7)	67,8 (±12.9)	
Male sex	50 (59.5)	5 (71.4)	45 (58.4)	0.5	40 (54.8)	10 (90.9)	0.023
Ethnicity							
White	76 (90.4)	6 (85.8)	70 (90.9)	0.654	68 (93.2)	8 (72.7)	0.031
Non-White	8 (9.6)	1 (14.2)	7 (9.1)	0.654	5 (6.8)	3 (27.3)	0.031
Index event							
Amourosis Fugax	14 (16.7)	3 (42.9)	11 (14.3)	0.052	14 (19.2)	0 (0)	0.11
TIA	31 (36.9)	3 (42.9)	28 (36.4)	0.73	26 (35.6)	5 (45.5)	0.53
Ischemic infarction	39 (46.4)	1 (14.2)	38 (49.3)	0.075	33 (45.2)	6 (54.5)	0.56
Carotid intervention							
CEA	29 (34.5)	4 (57.1)	25 (32.5)	0.19	26 (35.6)	3 (27.3)	0.59
Stent	19 (22.6)	0 (0)	19 (24.7)	0.135	17 (23.3)	2 (18.2)	0.71
History							
Stroke	32 (38.1)	3 (42.9)	29 (37.7)	0.79	27 (37.0)	5 (45.5)	0.59
Coronary Artery Disease	20 (23.8)	0 (0)	20 (26.0)	0.12	13 (17.8)	7 (63.6)	0.001
Peripheral Artery Disease	13 (15.5)	0 (0)	13 (16.9)	0.24	10 (13.7)	3 (27.3)	0.25
Risk Factors							
Current Smoker	35 (41.7)	3 (42.9)	32 (41.6)	0.95	29 (39.7)	6 (54.5)	0.35
Ex-smoker	30 (35.7)	3 (42.9)	27 (35.1)	0.68	28 (38.4)	2 (18.2)	0.19
Hypertension	60 (71.4)	4 (57.1)	56 (72.7)	0.38	50 (68.5)	10 (90.9)	0.13
Diabetes mellitus	22 (26.2)	0 (0)	22 (28.6)	0.10	16 (21.9)	6 (54.5)	0.022
Hypercholesteroleamia	51 (60.7)	3 (42.9)	48 (62.3)	0.31	41 (56.2)	10 (90.9)	0.028
Symptomatic Extracranial Stenosis							
0 - 29%	10 (11.9)	2 (28.7)	8 (10.4)	0.16	10 (13.7)	0 (0)	0.19

Table 1. (Continued)

Baseline characteristics		Intracranial internal carotid artery stenosis						
	Total	<30%	≥ 30%	p	<70%	≥ 70%	p
Symptomatic Extracranial Stenosis							
30 – 49%	9 (10.7)	1 (14.2)	8 (10.4)	0.75	9 (12.3)	0 (0)	0.22
50 – 69%	27 (32.1)	3 (42.9)	24 (31.2)	0.53	22 (30.1)	5 (45.5)	0.31
70 – 99%	30 (35.7)	1 (14.2)	29 (37.7)	0.23	25 (34.2)	5 (45.5)	0.47
Occlusion	8 (9.6)	0 (0)	8 (10.4)	0.37	7 (9.7)	1 (9.0)	0.96

Data are in mean ± standard deviation (SD) or number (n) of patients (%).

TIA = Transient Ischaemic Attack. CEA = Carotid Endarterectomy.

Table 2. the distribution of events in the follow-up period in patients with and without intracranial ICA stenosis (left part) and in patients with and without severe intracranial ICA stenosis (right part)

Follow-up	Intracranial internal carotid artery stenosis (n=84)					
	<30%	≥ 30%	OR (95% CI)	<70%	≥ 70%	OR (95% CI)
Event	n=7	n=77		n=73	n=11	
TIA	1 (14)	6 (8)	0.51 (0.05 - 4.93)	6 (8)	1 (9)	1.12 (0.12 - 10.27)
Cerebral Infarct	0 (0)	11 (14)	2.59 (0.14 - 48.6)	10 (14)	1 (9)	0.63 (0.07 - 5.5)
Myocardial Infarction	0 (0)	10 (13)	2.33 (0.12 - 43.9)	9 (12)	1 (9)	0.71 (0.08 - 6.23)
Vascular Death	0 (0)	12 (16)	2.86 (0.15 - 53.4)	7 (10)	5 (46)	7.85 (1.9 - 32.5)
Combined Endpoint	1 (14)	28 (36)	3.4 (0.39 - 30)	23 (32)	6 (55)	2.6 (0.72 - 9.43)
mRS ≥ 3	0 (0)	28 (36)	8.64 (0.48 - 157)	21 (29)	7 (64)	4.33 (1.15 - 16.37)

Data are in number (n) of events (%) or OR (95% CI).

OR = Odds Ratio.

TIA= Transient Ischaemic Attack.

mRS = modified Rankin Scale.

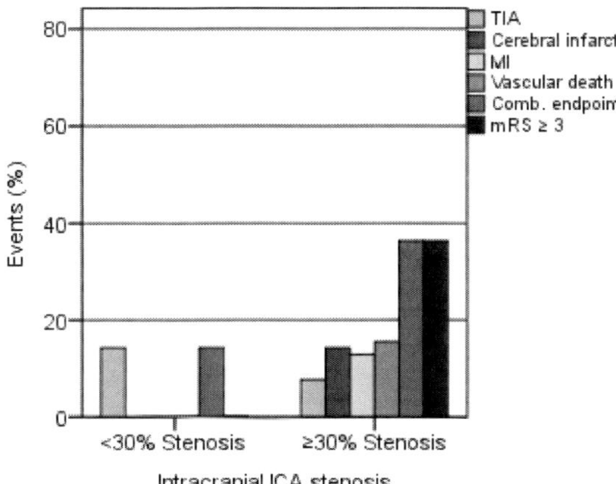

Figure 1. Bar chart of number of events (%) comparing patients without stenosis (<30%) to patients with stenosis (≥30%).

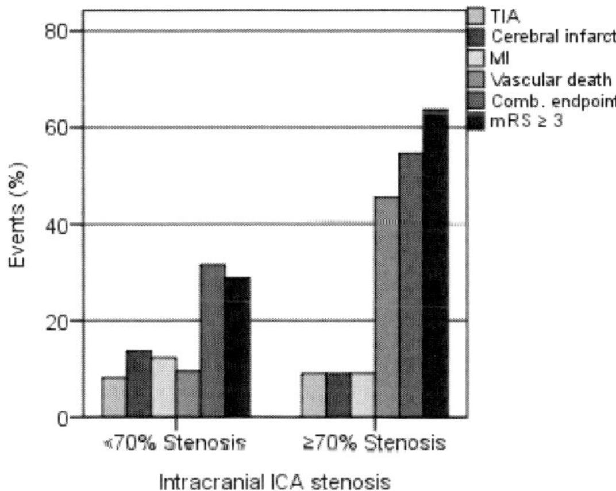

Figure 2. Bar chart of number of events (%) comparing patients without severe stenosis (<70%) to patients with severe stenosis (≥70%).

Twelve were regarded vascular deaths (16%) and all occurred in patients with any (≥30%) stenosis (OR 2.86 (0.15 - 53.4)).

Five of these deaths (46%) occurred in the group of patients with a severe stenosis (≥70%) (OR 7.85 (1.9 - 32.5)). Twenty-nine patients reached the combined endpoint of TIA, cerebral infarct, myocardial infarction, or vascular death.

One patient (14%) without any stenosis reached the combined endpoint, as compared with 28 patients (36%) with any stenosis (OR 3.4 (0.39 - 30)). Twenty-three patients (32%) without a severe stenosis reached the combined endpoint, as compared with 6 patients (55%) with a severe stenosis (OR 2.6 (0.72 - 9.43)). A total of 28 patients had a poor functional outcome (mRS ≥3). All of these patients had any intracranial stenosis. Twenty-one patients (29%) without a severe stenosis had a poor functional outcome, as compared with 7 patients (64%) with a severe stenosis (OR 4.33 (1.15 - 16.37)) (Table 2) (Figure 1 and 2). A Kaplan–Meier survival curve is shown in figure 3. This figure shows that the mortality rate is higher in patients with any intracranial ICA stenosis as compared with patients without any intracranial ICA stenosis, but this was not statistically significant (p=0.28)

Discussion

In this chapter we have shown that patients with any intracranial ICA stenosis (≥30%) on CTA images did not have a significantly higher rate of recurrent TIA, infarct or secondary outcomes compared to patients without stenosis (<30%). When comparing patients without severe stenosis (<70%) with patients with a severe stenosis (≥70%), also no increase in rate of recurrent TIA of infarct was found, but severe intracranial ICA stenosis was associated with vascular death and a poor functional outcome. In our previous study, we found that as much as 84% of the patients with extracranial internal carotid artery (ICA) stenosis and acute ischemic symptoms did also have an intracranial ICA stenosis in CT angiography data sets. We believe this prevalence is high as a result of the use of 64-section CTA for imaging.

In this previous study, we have also shown that the degree of extracranial ICA stenosis is not correlated with the degree of intracranial stenosis in this patient group. [9]

Present study shows that severe intracranial ICA stenosis (≥70%) is associated with male sex, non-white race, a history of ischemic heart disease, diabetes and hypercholesteroleamia. A previous analysis of the WASID cohort shows that diabetes and lipid disorder are associated with severity of intracranial stenosis, our study supports these findings. [11] This chapter also shows that diabetes was specifically associated with intracranial carotid artery stenosis, compared with other locations of intracranial stenosis, however, the pathological mechanism of this difference remains unclear.

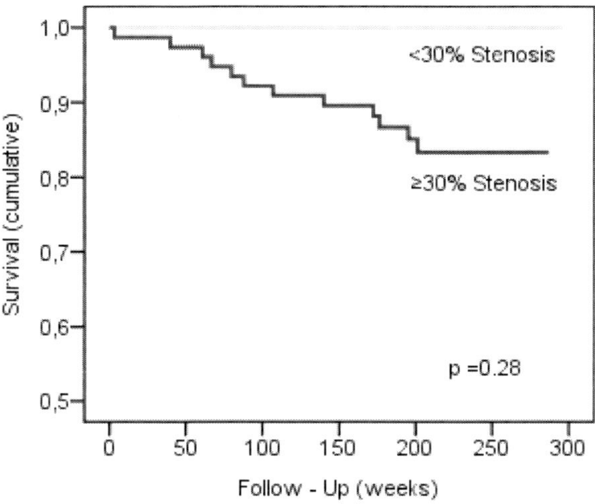

Figure 3. Kaplan-Meier analysis showing vascular death in patients with and without intracranial carotid artery stenosis.

Other studies show an association between male sex [5] and black race [14] and symptomatic intracranial stenosis, but an association between these risk factors and severity of intracranial ICA stenosis has not been reported before.

The rate of recurrent stroke in our current study (22%), 8% recurrent TIA and 14% cerebral infarct in patients with intracranial ICA stenosis, is comparable to previously reported 18% and 19% recurrent stroke in comparable cohorts. [4, 15] These studies, however, had shorter follow-up periods compared with present study. When comparing cardiovascular events during follow-up between the four subgroups, we found some remarkable results. Firstly, we found a difference in the number of events between patients with any stenosis, as compared with patients without any stenosis: only 1 event (TIA) occurred in 7 patients without any stenosis, whereas 39 events (TIA, infarct, myocardial infarction or vascular death) occurred in the 77 patients with any stenosis. Though this was not statistically significant, there is a clear trend that the presence of any intracranial ICA stenosis is associated with an increase of cardiovascular events during follow-up. Secondly, we found a clear association between the severity of intracranial ICA stenosis and functional outcome. The odds ratio for vascular death and poor functional outcome was significantly higher for patients with presence of severe intracranial ICA stenosis. The high number of vascular deaths may be due to the high number of patients with vascular risk factors in the group of patients with severe intracranial ICA stenosis. 91% of these patients had diabetes and hypercholesteroleamia and 64% had a history of coronary artery disease, all of these factors contribute to the risk of vascular death. An increase of vascular deaths in patients with intracranial ICA stenosis has been reported previously and our results support these findings. [16] The functional outcome, as measured on the modified Rankin Scale (mRS), in patients with severe stenosis, has to our knowledge not been reported before.

However, six of the seven patients with severe stenosis and a poor functional outcome were deaths. There was no increase in patients with severe disability (mRS = 4 or 5) in patients with severe intracranial stenosis (figure 4).

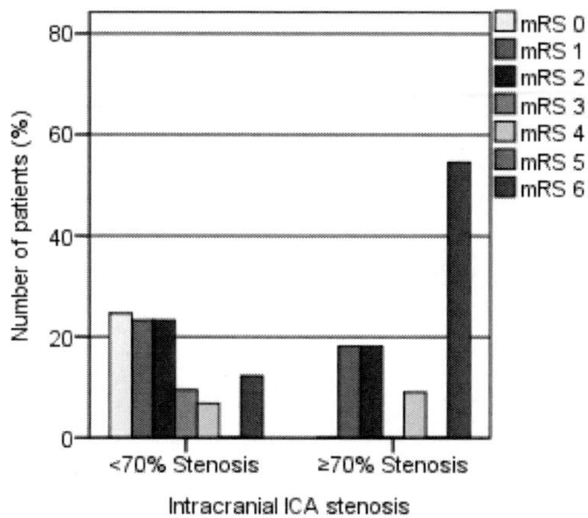

Figure 4. Modified Rankin Scale in patients without and with severe intracranial ICA stenosis.

We found a clear association between severe intracranial ICA stenosis and vascular death, however, we could not find such an association for the occurrence of recurrent TIA or stroke. This result was unexpected, as previous studies show a clear increase in risk of recurrent stroke in patients with intracranial stenosis, especially in patients with severe stenosis ($\geq$70%). [15, 17] Our results support a large study in a German population that concludes that there is no clear association between recurrent stroke and intracranial stenosis. [18] However, this study had a considerably lower prevalence of intracranial stenosis (6.5%) as compared with present study. An explanation for the difference may be the composition of the study population. Studies by

Kasner et al. and Wong et al. used a 42% non-white and Asian population, whereas the study by Weimar et al. and present study used a largely white population. The association between intracranial stenosis and recurrent stroke in a largely white population is less clear as compared with other populations. Considering the current risks of intracranial stenting, this association needs to be further evaluated. [19]

There are several limitations to our study. Patients were asked to recall events in a time span of 3 to 5 years.

As a result, events could have been missed, which results in an underestimation of the incidence of events. We limited this risk by collecting medical records of all patients, and by contacting the general practitioner in case of doubt. A second limitation to our study is the relatively small group size. The findings now need to be confirmed in a larger cohort with longer follow-up; in particular to investigate whether the risk of ipsilateral stroke is higher in patients with intracranial ICA stenosis.

Conclusion

Patients with any intracranial ICA stenosis did not have a significantly higher rate of recurrent TIA or infarct. Severe intracranial ICA stenosis on CTA in a white population is associated with a higher rate of vascular death and poor functional outcome. A larger prospective trial using CTA is needed to gain more insight on recurrent stroke rate and prevalence of intracranial ICA stenosis.

References

[1]   Lovett, J. K., Coull, A. J., Rothwell, P. M. Early risk of recurrence by subtype of ischemic stroke in population-based incidence studies. *Neurology.* 2004;62:569-573.

[2]   Khan, M., Naqvi, I., Bansari, A., Kamal, A. K. Intracranial atherosclerotic disease. *Stroke Res. Treat.* 2011;282845.

[3]   Arenillas, J. F. Intracranial atherosclerosis: current concepts. *Stroke.* 2011;42:S20-S23.

[4]   Kappelle, L. J., Eliasziw, M., Fox, A. J., Sharpe, B. L., Barnett, H. J. Importance of intracranial atherosclerotic disease in patients with

symptomatic stenosis of the internal carotid artery. The North American Symptomatic Carotid Endarterectomy Trail. *Stroke.* 1999;30:282-286.

[5]   Wityk, R. J., Lehman, D., Klag, M., Coresh, J., Ahn, H., Litt, B. Race and sex differences in the distribution of cerebral atherosclerosis. *Stroke.* 1996;27:1974-1980.

[6]   Nguyen-Huynh, M. N., Wintermark, M., English, J., et al. How accurate is CT angiography in evaluating intracranial atherosclerotic disease? *Stroke.* 2008;39:1184-1188.

[7]   Bash, S., Villablanca, J. P., Jahan, R., et al. Intracranial vascular stenosis and occlusive disease: evaluation with CT angiography, MR angiography, and digital subtraction angiography. *AJNR Am. J. Neuroradiol.* 2005;26:1012-1021.

[8]   Bleeker, L., Marquering, H. A., van den Berg, R., Nederkoorn, P. J., Majoie, C. B. Semi-automatic quantitative measurements of intracranial internal carotid artery stenosis and calcification using CT angiography. *Neuroradiology.* 2012;54:919-927.

[9]   Marquering, H. A., Nederkoorn, P. J., Bleeker, L., van den Berg, R., Majoie, C. B. Intracranial carotid artery disease in patients with recent neurological symptoms: high prevalence on CTA. *Neuroradiology.* 2013;55:179-85.

[10]   Samuels, O. B., Joseph, G. J., Lynn, M. J., Smith, H. A., Chimowitz, M. I. A standardized method for measuring intracranial arterial stenosis. *AJNR Am. J. Neuroradiol.* 2000;21:643-646.

[11]   Turan, T. N., Makki, A. A., Tsappidi, S., et al. Risk factors associated with severity and location of intracranial arterial stenosis. *Stroke.* 2010; 41:1636-1640.

[12]   Van Swieten, J. C., Koudstaal, P. J., Visser, M. C., Schouten, H. J., van Gijn, J. Interobserver agreement for the assessment of handicap in stroke patients. *Sitroke.* 1988;19:604-607.

[13]   Wilson, J. T., Hareendran, A., Grant, M., et al. Improving the assessment of outcomes in stroke: use of a structured interview to assign grades on the modified Rankin Scale. *Stroke.* 2002;33:2243-2246.

[14]   Sacco, R. L., Kargman, D. E., Zamanillo, M. C. Race-ethnic differences in stroke risk factors among hospitalized patients with cerebral infarction: the Northern Manhattan Stroke Study. *Neurology.* 1995;45: 659-663.

[15]   Kasner, S. E., Chimowitz, M. I., Lynn, M. J., et al. Predictors of ischemic stroke in the territory of a symptomatic intracranial arterial stenosis. *Circulation.* 2006;113:555-563.

[16] Klijn, C. J., Kappelle, L. J., Algra, A., van, G. J. Outcome in patients with symptomatic occlusion of the internal carotid artery or intracranial arterial lesions: a meta-analysis of the role of baseline characteristics and type of antithrombotic treatment. *Cerebrovasc. Dis.* 2001;12:228-234.

[17] Wong, K. S., Li, H. Long-term mortality and recurrent stroke risk among Chinese stroke patients with predominant intracranial atherosclerosis. *Stroke.* 2003;34:2361-2366.

[18] Weimar, C., Goertler, M., Harms, L., Diener, H. C. Distribution and outcome of symptomatic stenoses and occlusions in patients with acute cerebral ischemia. *Arch. Neurol.* 2006;63:1287-1291.

[19] Chimowitz, M. I., Lynn, M. J., Derdeyn, C. P., et al. Stenting versus aggressive medical therapy for intracranial arterial stenosis. *N. Engl. J. Med.* 2011;365:993-1003.

In: Carotid Artery Disease
Editor: Sherri Derricks

ISBN: 978-1-63321-859-8
© 2014 Nova Science Publishers, Inc.

Carotid Artery Atherosclerosis in Patients with Inflammatory Joint Diseases: Risk Factors, Prognosis and Management

S. Rollefstad, E. Ikdahl and A. G. Semb[*]
Preventive Cardio Rheuma clinic, Department of
Rheumatology, Diakonhjemmet Hospital, Oslo, Norway

Abstract

Patients with inflammatory joint diseases (IJD) have an increased risk of cardiovascular (CV) disease, which is of similar magnitude as for patients with diabetes; approximately twice as high as in the general population. Available CV risk calculators for the general population underestimate future CV events in patients with RA. The underestimation of CV risk may have several reasons:

---

[*] Corresponding author: A. G. Semb, MD, PhD. Leader, Preventive Cardio-Rheuma clinic, Department of Rheumatology, Diakonhjemmet Hospital, P.O. Box 23 Vinderen, NO-0319 Oslo, Norway. Tel: +47 91382216, fax: +47 22451777, e-mail: a-semb@diakonsyk.no.

1   systemic inflammation
2   a lipid paradox which has been described for patients with RA, whereby lower total cholesterol and low-density lipoprotein cholesterol were associated with increased risk of CV morbidity and mortality
3   the high frequency of asymptomatic carotid plaques (CP) in patients with RA.

In the recent European guidelines for CV disease prevention, CP is considered a very high CV disease risk factor; a CV disease equivalent. Therefore, it is recommended to initiate intensive lipid lowering treatment with statins when CP has been identified in a patient. Thus it is important to identify CP.

Introduction

Patients with inflammatory joint diseases (IJD) have an increased risk of cardiovascular (CV) disease. Within the IJD group, patients with rheumatoid arthritis (RA) have been most extensively investigated concerning CV risk [1, 2], but the CV burden of patients with psoriatic arthritis (PsA) [3, 4] and ankylosing spondylitis (AS) [5, 6] has also been documented to be increased compared to the general population. The CV risk for patients with RA is of similar magnitude as for patients with diabetes [1, 7], which is approximately twice as high as in the general population. Thus, enhancement of CV risk evaluation in patients with IJD has been called upon [8].

Available CV risk calculators for the general population underestimate future CV events in patients with RA [9, 10]. The underestimation of CV risk may have several reasons and can be related to systemic inflammation and to a lipid paradox which has been described for patients with RA, whereby lower total cholesterol and low-density lipoprotein cholesterol (LDL-c) were associated with increased risk of CV morbidity and mortality [11].

Another reason may be the high frequency of asymptomatic carotid plaques (CP) in patients with RA [12-15]. Indeed, the presence of CP in RA patients has been shown to predict future acute coronary syndromes [16]. If CP were bilaterally present, the risk of acute coronary syndrome was quadrupled. In accordance with this, Ajeganova and colleagues found an association between bilateral CP and poor CV disease outcome [17]. In the recent European guidelines for CV disease prevention [18], CP is considered a very high CV disease risk factor; a CV disease equivalent. Therefore, it is recommended to initiate intensive lipid lowering treatment with statins when CP has been identified in a patient. Thus it is important to identify CP.

An inexpensive and non-invasive method to do so is B-Mode ultrasound of the carotid arteries. Consequently, if ultrasound of carotid arteries is included as a part of the CV risk evaluation in patients with IJD, the proportion of patients categorized to the correct CV risk group will increase [19, 20]. Aspects of carotid artery atherosclerosis in patients with IJD including risk factors, prognosis and management will be discussed.

Ultrasound of the Carotid Arteries

Bilateral B-mode carotid ultrasonography examinations may be performed in accordance to published recommendations [21], using a 9-14 MHz linear matrix array transducer. Intima-media thickness (IMT) can be measured in the far wall (FW) of the common carotid artery (CCA) over a 5 mm long segment, from approximately 10 mm proximal to the start of the carotid bulb (bulb). It is necessary that both near wall and FW of the artery are visualized with sharp edges (indicating an isonation of about 90° to the vessel wall) before images are stored for analysis, to avoid overestimation of IMT and plaque size. Atherosclerotic plaques in the CCA, bulb and the internal carotid artery can be identified in the longitudinal view as protrusions into the lumen > 1.5 mm, or at least 2 times the adjacent IMT. The presence of a plaque should be verified by a cross sectional image obtained by rotating the probe 90°.

Patients with RA Have Twice As Many CP As People without RA

A study involving 152 RA patients and 89 controls showed that RA patients had a higher frequency of CP, which were also more often bilaterally present compared to controls (age and gender adjusted) [14]. From a preventive cardio-rheuma clinic it is reported that CP were present in almost half of the patients who underwent CV risk evaluation, and these patients had a median disease duration of more than 10 years [15]. Although, results from a very early RA cohort revealed no higher frequency of atherosclerosis compared to controls in the initial phase of the joint disease [22]. However, in this study markers of accelerated atherosclerosis, such as endothelial dysfunction (measured by flow mediated dilation) and increased IMT, were found to be more prevalent in patients with early RA compared to controls.

Eder et al. have reported that in patients with PsA (n=40), compared to 40 matched controls, there was a higher prevalence of CP amongst the PsA patients, and also more severe plaques measured by grade of stenosis [23].

Risk Factors of Carotid Atherosclerosis in Patients with IJD

The etiology of the high prevalence of carotid atherosclerosis may include both genetic and environmental factors. Risk factors for development of carotid atherosclerosis such as age, smoking, obesity, hypercholesterolemia and hypertension are described for the general population [24]. It is not exclusively the presence of CP, but also the plaque vulnerability to rupture which is associated with CV events. Autopsy studies have suggested that RA patients have more inflammatory and unstable coronary artery plaques compared to controls [12]. It has also been demonstrated that patients with RA have different carotid wall remodeling (the change of the arterial wall structural properties in response to hemodynamic or metabolic factors) compared to healthy controls, with widening of the arterial diameter resulting in increased wall stress and tension, possibly contributing to plaque instability and rupture [25]. In addition, it has been shown that women with RA have increased carotid artery diameter compared with healthy women, indicating a premature aging of the arteries [26]. In a study exploring the association of joint disease activity and plaque vulnerability, patients with active RA disease (assessed by the Clinical Disease Activity Index) had more vulnerable CP than patients in remission [14]. These findings suggest that remission is the mission not only for the rheumatic joint disease but also for prevention of CV disease.

Predictors of Progression of Carotid Atherosclerosis in RA

Giles and colleagues performed a longitudinal study which aimed to explore possible predictors of progression of carotid atherosclerosis in patients with RA without documented CV disease prior to study inclusion [27]. Higher levels of systemic inflammation (measured by cumulative average CRP) and swollen joint counts were found to be associated with progression of CP present at baseline, or with development of CP during the study period.

Furthermore, results from the discussed study indicate that patients early in the RA disease course had accelerated progression of carotid atherosclerosis compared to patients at a later stage of the joint disease.

A possible explanation for these findings may be a higher inflammatory burden early in the disease. In addition, a survival effect could be applicable meaning that patients with the longest disease duration, who have had a rapid progression of atherosclerosis, may also have experienced a CV event earlier in the joint disease course which was an exclusion criterion for the study.

Ultrasound of Carotid Arteries Enhances Correct CV Risk Evaluation in Patients with IJD

Markers of preclinical atherosclerosis, such as endothelial dysfunction, arterial stiffness, increased IMT and presence of CP, are as common in RA patients compared to those having diabetes, suggesting that the excess CV risk should be addressed as aggressively in RA as in diabetes [13]. However, CV risk algorithms developed for the general population are poor predictors of CP.

CV risk evaluation in IJD patients (n= 335) was performed using the Systematic Coronary Risk Evaluation (SCORE) algorithm. Carotid ultrasound contributed to correct CV risk classification in about 45 % of IJD patients calculated by SCORE to have a low or moderate risk, and 60 % of IJD patients with high risk of future CV events, with initiation of recommended intensive lipid lowering treatment (LLT) as the clinical consequence. Optimizing the CV risk cut off level for indication of LLT by 2 validated methods yielded an improvement in number of patients classified into intensive LLT, although an unacceptable number of patients with CP (20-30 %) were still classified to no or inadequate LLT [19].

Recommendations for CV risk assessment in patients with RA and other forms of inflammatory joint diseases have been published [28]. These recommendations suggests that in RA patients fulfilling at least 2 out of 3 of the following criteria: disease duration >10 years, rheumatoid factor/anticitrullinated protein antibody positivity, or extra-articular manifestations, the calculated CV risk should be multiplied by 1.5.

The multiplication factor was derived mainly from relevant standardized mortality ratios, because information from large-scale prospective cohort studies is lacking.

However, Corrales et al. have shown that the discussed multiplication factor only reclassifies 0.03% of the patients into more appropriate CV disease risk classes, but even then patients at high risk and those with asymptomatic carotid atherosclerosis were not adequately identified. Hence, the 1.5 multiplication factor does not adjust for the increased risk of CV disease in RA [29].

Will Prophylactic Treatment with Statins Reduce the Risk of Atherosclerotic Plaque-Related Events in Patients with RA?

The evidence is scarce concerning the effect of statins on the morphology of CP in patients with RA. However, we have conducted a trial on the effect of intensive statin treatment on change in CP size [30, 31].

In the ROsuvastatin in Rheumatoid Arthritis, Ankylosing Spondylitis and other inflammatory joint diseases (RORA-AS) study, the aims were to evaluate change in CP, and whether laboratory values or clinical indicators were predictors of the potential change in CP after 18 months of intensive LLT. The RORA-AS study was a prospective, open intervention study where 86 statin naïve patients with IJD (RA n=55, AS n=21, PsA n=10) and CP who were treated with rosuvastatin to obtain a LDL-c goal $\leq$1.8 mmol/L. Carotid ultrasound was performed at baseline and after 18 months to evaluate the CP height.

Compliance of rosuvastatin was 97.9%. Intensive treatment with rosuvastatin induced CP height regression and reduced LDL-c significantly in patients with IJD. The LDL-c goal attainment, the change in LDL-c or the LDL-c level exposure during the study period did not influence the degree of CP height reduction. Prospective randomized statin studies with clinical endpoints are warranted to reveal if height reduction of asymptomatic CP will have impact on future CV events.

References

[1] Lindhardsen, J., Ahlehoff, O., Gislason, G. H., Madsen, O. R., Olesen, J. B., Torp-Pedersen, C., Hansen, P. R. The risk of myocardial infarction in rheumatoid arthritis and diabetes mellitus: a Danish nationwide cohort study. *Ann. Rheum. Dis.* 2011, 70, 929-34.

[2] Aviña-Zubieta, J. A., Choi, H. K., Sadatsafavi, M., Etminan, M., Esdaile, J. M., Lacaille, D. Risk of cardiovascular mortality in patients with rheumatoid arthritis: a meta-analysis of observational studies. *Arthritis Rheum.* 2008, 59, 1690-7.

[3] Han, C., Robinson, D. W. Jr, Hackett, M. V., Paramore, L. C., Fraeman, K. H., Bala, M. V. Cardiovascular disease and risk factors in patients with rheumatoid arthritis, psoriatic arthritis, and ankylosing spondylitis. *J. Rheumatol.* 2006, 33, 2167-72.

[4] Tobin, A. M., Veale, D. J., Fitzgerald, O., Rogers, S., Collins, P., O'Shea, D., Kirby, B. Cardiovascular disease and risk factors in patients with psoriasis and psoriatic arthritis. *J. Rheumatol.* 2010, 37, 1386-94.

[5] Peters, M. J., van der Horst-Bruinsma, I. E., Dijkmans, B. A., Nurmohamed, M. T. Cardiovascular risk profile of patients with spondylarthropathies, particularly ankylosing spondylitis and psoriatic arthritis. *Semin. Arthritis Rheum.* 2004, 34, 585-92.

[6] Peters, M. J., van Eijk, I. C., Smulders, Y. M., Serne, E., Dijkmans, B. A., van der Horst-Bruinsma, I. E., Nurmohamed, M. T. Signs of accelerated preclinical atherosclerosis in patients with ankylosing spondylitis. *J. Rheumatol.* 2010, 37, 161-6.

[7] Van Halm, V. P., Peters, M. J., Voskuyl, A. E., Boers, M., Lems, W. F., Visser, M., Stehouwer, C. D., Spijkerman, A. M., Dekker, J. M., Nijpels, G., Heine, R. J., Bouter, L. M., Smulders, Y. M., Dijkmans, B. A., Nurmohamed, M. T. Rheumatoid arthritis versus diabetes as a risk factor for cardiovascular disease: a cross-sectional study, the CARRE Investigation. *Ann. Rheum. Dis.* 2009, 68, 1395-400.

[8] Semb, A. G., Rollefstad, S., van Riel, P., Kitas, G. D., Matteson, E. L., Gabriel, S. E. Cardiovascular disease assessment in rheumatoid arthritis: a guide to translating knowledge of cardiovascular risk into clinical practice. *Ann. Rheum. Dis.* 2014, 73,1284-8.

[9] Crowson, C. S., Matteson, E. L., Roger, V. L., Therneau, T. M., Gabriel, S. E. Usefulness of risk scores to estimate the risk of cardiovascular

disease in patients with rheumatoid arthritis. *Am. J. Cardiol.* 2012, 110, 420-4.

[10] Arts, E. E., Popa, C., Den Broeder, A. A., Semb, A. G., Toms, T., Kitas, G. D., van Riel, P. L., Fransen, J. Performance of four current risk algorithms in predicting cardiovascular events in patients with early rheumatoid arthritis. *Ann. Rheum. Dis.* 2014, doi: 10.1136/annrheumdis-2013-204024.

[11] Myasoedova, E., Crowson, C. S., Kremers, H. M., Roger, V. L., Fitz-Gibbon, P. D., Therneau, T. M., Gabriel, S. E. Lipid paradox in rheumatoid arthritis: the impact of serum lipid measures and systemic inflammation on the risk of cardiovascular disease. *Ann. Rheum. Dis.* 2011, 70, 482-7.

[12] Roman, M. J., Moeller, E., Davis, A., Paget, S. A., Crow, M. K., Lockshin, M. D., Sammaritano, L., Devereux, R. B., Schwartz, J. E., Levine, D. M., Salmon, J. E. Preclinical carotid atherosclerosis in patients with rheumatoid arthritis. *Ann. Intern. Med.* 2006, 144, 249-56.

[13] Stamatelopoulos, K. S., Kitas, G. D., Papamichael, C. M., Chryssohoou, E., Kyrkou, K., Georgiopoulos, G., Protogerou, A., Panoulas, V. F., Sandoo, A., Tentolouris, N., Mavrikakis, M., Sfikakis, P. P. Atherosclerosis in rheumatoid arthritis versus diabetes: a comparative study. *Arterioscler. Thromb. Vasc. Biol.* 2009, 29, 1702-8.

[14] Semb, A. G., Rollefstad, S., Provan, S. A., Kvien, T. K., Stranden, E., Olsen, I. C., Hisdal, J. Carotid plaque characteristics and disease activity in rheumatoid arthritis. *J. Rheumatol.* 2013, 40, 359-68.

[15] Rollefstad, S., Kvien, T. K., Holme, I., Eirheim, A. S., Pedersen, T. R., Semb, A. G. Treatment to lipid targets in patients with inflammatory joint diseases in a preventive cardio-rheuma clinic. *Ann. Rheum. Dis.* 2013, 72, 1968-74.

[16] Evans, M. R., Escalante, A., Battafarano, D. F., Freeman, G. L., O'Leary, D. H., del Rincón, I. Carotid atherosclerosis predicts incident acute coronary syndromes in rheumatoid arthritis. *Arthritis Rheum.* 2011, 63, 1211-20.

[17] Ajeganova, S., de Faire, U., Jogestrand, T., Frostegård, J., Hafström, I. Carotid atherosclerosis, disease measures, oxidized low-density lipoproteins, and atheroprotective natural antibodies for cardiovascular disease in early rheumatoid arthritis -- an inception cohort study. *J. Rheumatol.* 2012, 39, 1146-54.

[18] Perk, J., De Backer, G., Gohlke, H., Graham, I., Reiner, Z., Verschuren, M., Albus, C., Benlian, P., Boysen, G., Cifkova, R., Deaton, C.,

Ebrahim, S., Fisher, M., Germano, G., Hobbs, R., Hoes, A., Karadeniz, S., Mezzani, A., Prescott, E., Ryden, L., Scherer, M., Syvänne, M., Scholte op Reimer, W. J., Vrints, C., Wood, D., Zamorano, J. L., Zannad, F.; European Association for Cardiovascular Prevention and Rehabilitation (EACPR); ESC Committee for Practice Guidelines (CPG). European Guidelines on cardiovascular disease prevention in clinical practice (version 2012). The Fifth Joint Task Force of the European Society of Cardiology and Other Societies on Cardiovascular Disease Prevention in Clinical Practice (constituted by representatives of nine societies and by invited experts). *Eur. Heart J.* 2012, 33, 1635-701.

[19] Semb, A. G., Rollefstad, S., Hisdahl, J., Ikdahl, E., Eirheim, A. S., Heijde, D. van der, Kvien, T. K., Olsen, I.C. Ultrasound of carotid arteries enhances correct cardiovascular risk evaluation in patients with inflammatory joint diseases. *Rheumatol.* (Oxford) 2014 (in press).

[20] Corrales, A., González-Juanatey, C., Peiró, M. E., Blanco, R., Llorca, J., González-Gay, M. A. Carotid ultrasound is useful for the cardiovascular risk stratification of patients with rheumatoid arthritis: results of a population-based study. *Ann. Rheum. Dis.* 2014, 73, 722-7.

[21] Roman, M. J., Naqvi, T. Z., Gardin, J. M., Gerhard-Herman, M., Jaff, M., Mohler, E. Clinical application of noninvasive vascular ultrasound in cardiovascular risk stratification: a report from the American Society of Echocardiography and the Society of Vascular Medicine and Biology. *J. Am. Soc. Echocardiogr.* 2006, 19, 943-954.

[22] Södergren, A., Karp, K., Boman, K., Eriksson, C., Lundström, E., Smedby, T., Söderlund, L., Rantapää-Dahlqvist, S., Wållberg-Jonsson, S. Atherosclerosis in early rheumatoid arthritis: very early endothelial activation and rapid progression of intima media thickness. *Arthritis Res. Ther.* 2010, 12, R158.

[23] Eder, L., Zisman, D., Barzilai, M., Laor, A., Rahat, M., Rozenbaum, M., Bitterman, H., Feld, J., Rimar, D., Rosner, I. Subclinical atherosclerosis in psoriatic arthritis: a case-control study. *J. Rheumatol.* 2008, 35, 877-82.

[24] Kang, S., Wu, Y., Li, X. Effects of statin therapy on the progression of carotid atherosclerosis: a systematic review and meta-analysis. *Atherosclerosis* 2004, 177, 433-42.

[25] Van Sijl, A. M., Van Den Hurk, K., Peters, M. J., Van Halm, V. P., Nijpels, G., Stehouwer, C. D., Smulders, Y. V., Voskuyl, A. E., Dekker, J. M., Nurmohamed, M. T. Different type of carotid arterial wall

remodeling in rheumatoid arthritis compared with healthy subjects: a case-control study. *J. Rheumatol.* 2012, 39, 2261-6.

[26] Schott, L. L., Kao, A. H., Cunningham, A., Wildman, R. P., Kuller, L. H., Sutton-Tyrrell, K., Wasko, M. C. Do carotid artery diameters manifest early evidence of atherosclerosis in women with rheumatoid arthritis? *J. Womens Health* (Larchmt). 2009, 18, 21-9.

[27] Giles, J. T., Post, W. S., Blumenthal, R. S., Polak, J., Petri, M., Gelber, A. C., Szklo, M., Bathon, J. M. Longitudinal predictors of progression of carotid atherosclerosis in rheumatoid arthritis. *Arthritis Rheum.* 2011, 63, 3216-25.

[28] Peters, M. J., Symmons, D. P., McCarey, D., Dijkmans, B. A., Nicola, P., Kvien, T. K., McInnes, I. B., Haentzschel, H., Gonzalez-Gay, M. A., Provan, S., Semb, A., Sidiropoulos, P., Kitas, G., Smulders, Y. M., Soubrier, M., Szekanecz, Z., Sattar, N., Nurmohamed, M. T. EULAR evidence-based recommendations for cardiovascular risk management in patients with rheumatoid arthritis and other forms of inflammatory arthritis. *Ann. Rheum. Dis.* 2010, 69, 325-31.

[29] Corrales, A., Parra, J. A., González-Juanatey, C., Rueda-Gotor, J., Blanco, R., Llorca, J., González-Gay, M. A. Cardiovascular risk stratification in rheumatic diseases: carotid ultrasound is more sensitive than Coronary Artery Calcification Score to detect subclinical atherosclerosis in patients with rheumatoid arthritis. *Ann. Rheum. Dis.* 2013, 72, 1764-70.

[30] http://clinicaltrials.gov/ct2/show/NCT01389388?term=Rosuvastatin+and +rheumatoid+Arthritisandrank=3.

[31] Rollefstad, S., Ikdahl, E., Hisdal, J., Olsen, I. C., Smerud, K. T., Kitas, G. D., Pedersen, T. R., Kvien, T. K., Semb, A. G. Rosuvastatin induced carotid plaque regression in patients with inflammatory joint diseases. *Ann. Rheum. Dis.* 2014;73(Suppl. 2).

In: Carotid Artery Disease
Editor: Sherri Derricks

ISBN: 978-1-63321-859-8
© 2014 Nova Science Publishers, Inc.

Chapter 4

The Impact of Obesity on Carotid Artery Disease in Obese Adolescents

Raquel Munhoz da Silveira Campos,*
Ana Raimunda Dâmaso
and Deborah Cristina Landi Masquio
Universidade Federal de São Paulo (UNIFESP),
Post-Graduate Program of Nutrition, São Paulo-SP, Brasil

Abstract

Obesity is a multifactorial disease, characterized by excessive body fat accumulation, which is increasing worldwide in all age. Excessive body fat is related to a chronic inflammation due to the pro-inflammatory adipokines secreted mainly by visceral fat. Additionally, this inflammation is related to cardiometabolic alterations, such as insulin resistance, dyslipidemia, hypertension, hyperleptinemia, metabolic syndrome and non-alcoholic fatty liver disease, which potentiate Accessed June cardiovascular risks, such as increase in carotid intima media thickness (cIMT), including in adolescence. The present chapter aims to review the role of obesity and its comorbidities on carotid artery

* Corresponding author's email: raquelmunhoz@hotmail.com.

disease in obese adolescents, and the main effects of physical exercise and nutrition. Carotid Intima media thickness (cIMT) is considered an important method of estimating early subclinical signal of atherosclerosis process. An increase of carotid artery is a result from endothelial dysfunction that creates lipid deposits in the intima media of systemic arteries. Such deposits can be caused by inflammation, metabolic alterations and saturated fatty acid intake. The exposure during childhood to these metabolic alterations may contribute to the development of atherosclerosis. In obese adolescents, insulin resistance, visceral fat, leptin/adiponectin ratio and PAI-1 concentration were positive associated with cIMT. Additionally, the diet can also influence carotid artery in obese patients. Saturated fatty acids can predict cIMT, and every 10g of saturated fatty intake per day was associated with increase of 0.03 mm on cIMT. On the other hand, interdisciplinary intervention has been effective in reducing cIMT in obese adolescents with comorbidities, such as metabolic syndrome, non-alcoholic fatty liver disease, hyperleptinemia and insulin resistance. Moreover, reduction in 10% of weight loss can contribute in cIMT reduction in obese adolescents. In conclusion, obesity and metabolic disorders appeared to explain increase of carotid artery disorders, enhancing cardiovascular risks. However, interdisciplinary therapy, including nutritional interventions and physical exercise, may prevent and control obesity related comorbidities, associated with a control of increase in cIMT in obese adolescents.

Introduction

Obesity is characterized as a chronic disease related to several comorbidities that lead to the development of cardiovascular disease. The prevalence of this disease is increasing worldwide, in all ages, which arises concerns about its impact on quality of life. The obesity etiology is multifactorial and includes mainly sedentary and eating habits, which are the two major modifiable lifestyle factors included in its treatment (WHO, 2014).

The low-grade inflammatory state observed in obesity is associated with the excessive visceral fat located in abdominal region. Concomitantly, the increase of pro-inflammatory adipokines and the reduction of anti-inflammatory adipokines can lead to metabolic alterations, such as, insulin resistance, dyslipidemia and hypertension. This constellation of metabolic alteration is defined as metabolic syndrome. Moreover, metabolic syndrome potentiates cardiovascular disease development. Concomitantly, the adipokines secreted by visceral fat also present a key role in the development of carotid artery disease. In this way, metabolic alterations and inflammation are the main factors related to cardiovascular disease in obesity, even in adolescents (Fuentes et al., 2013).

Increased carotid intima media thickness (cIMT) is considered the first subclinical sign of atherosclerosis, resulting from endothelial dysfunction. Insulin resistance, inflammation, body weight and excessive saturated fatty acid intake can contribute to development of carotid artery disease. In this way, interdisciplinary approach to control obesity and its comorbidities has been demonstrated as an important strategy to prevent cardiovascular risks, including physical exercise and nutritional approach (Dâmaso et al. 2013, Masquio et al., 2013; Sanches et al., 2013). Thus, the present chapter will review the role of obesity and its comorbidities on carotid artery disease in obese adolescents, and the main effects of physical exercise and nutrition intervention in controlling this process.

Obesity: Definition, Etiology and Consequences

Overweight and obesity are defined as abnormal or excessive fat accumulation that may impair health (WHO, 2014). Adipose tissue is considered a potent source of hormones, peptides, and cytokines involved in food intake regulation, glucose and lipid metabolism, inflammation, coagulation and blood pressure control. Since adipose tissue was considered a secretory organ, obesity was defined as an inflammatory disease due to the increased secretion of pro-inflammatory adipokines (Fuentes et al., 2013).

In this way, obesity is associated with a chronic inflammatory response characterized by abnormal adipokines production and the activation of several proinflammatory signaling pathways, resulting in the induction of several biological markers of inflammation. Indeed, inflammation is receiving increased attention for its potential role in the pathogenesis of metabolic disorders, ranging from insulin resistance to fatty liver and cardiovascular diseases (Piya et al., 2013).

There are numerous adverse effects of overweight and obesity on general and cardiovascular health. In addition to squeal later in life, childhood obesity also has showed acute consequences during childhood. Most notably, obesity associated disorders are dyslipidemia, hypertension, non-alchoolic fatty liver disease, type 2 diabetes, obstructive sleep apnea, polycystic ovarian syndrome, infertility, orthopedic complications, psychiatric disease and cancer (Lavie et al., 2014, Kelsey et al., 2014).

Nowadays, obesity is a major public health concern, since excess bodyweight is an important risk factor for mortality and morbidity from cardiovascular diseases, diabetes and cancers, causing nearly three million deaths every year worldwide (Finucane et al., 2011; WHO, 2014). Additionally, the estimated annual medical cost of obesity in the U.S. was $147 billion U.S. dollars in 2008. Per capita, medical outlay for the obese is $1,429 per year, or roughly 42 percent higher than for a normal weight person (Eric et al., 2009). Moreover, in the last decades, obesity has increased in epidemic proportions in both adults and children (WHO, 2014). According to World Health Organization, 35% of adults aged 20+ were overweight, and the worldwide prevalence of obesity has nearly doubled between 1980 and 2008. More than 40 million children under the age of 5 were overweight or obese in 2012. Moreover, the prevalence of childhood overweight and obesity in preschool children is in excess of 30% (WHO, 2014). In Brazil, the prevalence of excessive weight in adolescents increased in the last three decades, reaching, 21.7% of boys and 19.4% of girls. In adults, nearby 50% of men and women are overweight (IBGE, 2010, Ministério da Saúde, 2014).

Although individual and genetic factors influence weight, the main cause of obesity is an energy imbalance between calories consumed and calories expended (Figure 1).

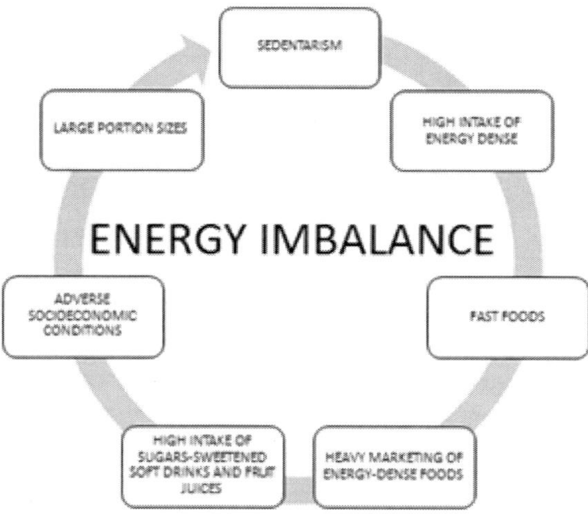

Figure 1. Factors that might promote weight gain and obesity. *Adapted from WHO, 2003.*

Globally, the increased intake of energy-dense foods that are high in fat and high glycemic index plus an increase in physical inactivity contribute for obesity and chronic disease development (WHO, 2003, Egger et al., 2014). For this reason, changes in diet and physical activity patterns are often the key management for obesity prevention and treatment (WHO, 2014).

Obesity and Inflammation

Obesity is an inflammatory state received important attention over the past 15 years. In particular, visceral fat seems to play an important endocrine role in the process of systemic inflammation in this population (de Ferranti et al., 2008). The excess lipid stores, especially in the visceral adipocytes, promote an increase of inflammatory adipokines such as tumor necrosis factor-α and interleukin-6 (Tilg H et al., 2008). These chemokines, in turn, promote the migration of macrophages to the adipose tissue, greatly increasing cytokine release (DeBoer, 2013; Giordano et al., 2013).

The term adipokines is used for any substance released by adipose tissue (Fain et al., 2004). In recent years, the number of adipokines has expanded rapidly and these also include adiponectin, resistin, visfatin, apelin, plasminogen activator inhibitor-1, tumor necrosis factor-α and interleukin-6 (Leal et al., 2013) (Table 1) (Figure 2).

It is important to note that, in obesity, the systemic inflammation appears to be associated with reduction of adiponectin adipokine, which is secreted by adipocytes in inverse proportion to the amount of stored lipid and appears to confer insulin sensitivity in animal models of obesity (Yamauchi et al., 2001; Lee et al., 2006). These low levels of adiponectin and increasing insulin resistance are also associated with the clinical features of metabolic syndrome (Ford et al., 2007; Zimmet et al., 2007). It was showed that low levels of adiponectin are associated with higher levels of inflammatory cytokines, whereas infusions of adiponectin in animal models result in a decrease in systemic inflammation; however the mechanisms are still unclear (Yamauchi et al., 2001). The secretory function of adipocytes can also be modulated by adipokines, as shown mainly in vitro models. TNF-α is known to suppress adiponectin production by adipocytes, while it induces a number of proinflammatory mediators like IL-6, MCP-1 and PAI-1 (Cawthorn and Sethi, 2008). IL-6 acts as a negative regulator of visfatin expression in 3T3L1 adipocytes (Kralisch et al., 2005) and does not alter leptin release (Bruun et al., 2002). The release of proinflammatory cytokines, TNF-α and IL-6, is also induced by resistin in isolated human subcutaneous adipocytes, an effect that seems to be possibly mediated by the NF-kB and JNK pathways (Kusminski et al., 2007).

Table 1. The role of principal pro-anti-inflammatory adipokines involve in obesity disease

LEPTIN	The principal biologic effect of leptin is the control of adipose tissue growth via its central nervous system (CNS) action. Leptin reduces appetite and increases energy expenditure.
ADIPONECTIN	Its actions are related to improvement of insulin sensitivity through activation of AMP protein kinase (AMPK) in liver and skeletal muscle and reduction of the hepatic gluconeogenesis enzyme expression. Adiponectin is inversely associated with the adhesion molecule expression and the transformation of macrophages into foam cells.
PLASMINOGEN ACTIVATOR INHIBITOR-1	PAI-1 is responsible for decreased fibrinolytic capacity and is consequently considered a cardiovascular risk factor.
RESISTIN	Resistin increases gluconeogenic enzymes expression in liver and decreases AMPK activity and insulin receptor substrate (IRS)-2 expressions.
APELIN	Apelin increases the activity of sarcolemmal Na+/H+-exchanger, leading to a positive inotropic effect without inducing myocardial hypertrophy.
VISFATIN	Visfatin appears atherogenic because it contributes to leukocyte adhesion and atherogenic plaque instability and may have a direct role in vascular dysfunction and inflammation through iNOS.
TUMOR NECROSIS FACTOR-α	It appears related to insulin resistance in skeletal muscle and adipose tissue due to abnormal phosphorylation of IRS-1 and decreased signal transduction for GLUT-4 translocation.
INTERLEUKIN-6	IL-6 is a proinflammatory factor produced by monocytes, fibroblasts and the stromal vascular fraction of visceral white adipose tissue. IL-6 induces liver production of C-reactive protein (CRP), an independent and important risk marker for cardiovascular disease.

CNS: central nervous system; AMPK: AMP protein kinase; PAI-1: Plasminogen Activator Inhibitor-1; IRS: insulin receptor substrate; CRP: C-reactive protein; IL-6: Interleukin-6. *Adapted from DeBoer, 2013.*

In addition, in obesity, hyperphagia and increased adipose mass in the presence of hyperleptinemia indicate a resistance to endogenous leptin (Vázquez-Vela et al., 2008; Coppari and Bjorbaek, 2012).

This constellation of pro-anti-inflammatory biomarkers secretion by excess visceral adipose is associated with central obesity and development of many comorbities including cardiovascular diseases (DeBoer, 2013) (Table 1 and Figure 2).

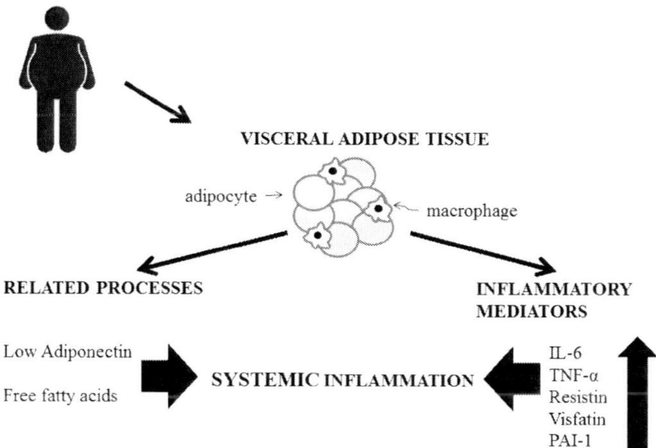

Figure 2. Effects of visceral adipose tissue expansion in obesity. Systemic Inflammation is characterized by an increase in pro-inflammatory mediators and related processes.

Obesity, Comorbidities and Cardiovascular Risk Factors

Obesity is characterized by excess of fat accumulation in adipose tissue in association with low pro-inflammatory state. The etiology is multifactorial and the mostly causes of obesity was associated with higher diet ingest and lower physical exercise activity, factors that contribute to a positive energetic balance. Moreover, environmental factors, cultural, psychology, genetic and others pathologies could be associated with obesity development. Nowadays, obesity is considerate a global epidemic with alarming numbers in the population. Moreover, the predictions show 2030 is that this number reaches more than 1 billion people, in addition are the development of many comorbidities such as non-alcoholic fatty liver, metabolic syndrome, dyslipidemia and diabetes mellitus.

Non-Alcoholic Fatty Liver Disease

Non-Alcoholic Fatty Liver Disease (NAFLD) is a commonly comorbidity observed in obesity individuals. Occurs in all age groups and can be present in any ethnicity. It was recognized clinically only in the 50s and characterized histologically in 1980 (Adams and Angulo, 2006). Prevalence data demonstrate the continuing and increasing incidence of this comorbidity in the population. It affects approximately 24% of the adult population but when these data are transferred to individuals with obesity, the prevalence reaches 74% and up to 90% of obese grade III (Tock et al., 2006; Lam and Younossi, 2010). The NAFLD affects a broad spectrum of tissue changes of the hepatocyte, ranging from simple steatosis to steatohepatitis and may even evolve into cirrhosis (Lam and Younossi, 2010). Approximately 5% of patients with NAFLD develop cirrhosis and only 2% can progress to death (Adams et al., 2005).

Physiologically, in the NAFLD, the fat accumulation is the result of increased influx of free fatty acids in the liver, increased lipogenesis exceeding the β-oxidation of fatty acids and exported of very low-density lipoprotein cholesterol (VLDL), causing hepatic fat accumulation (Dowman et al., 2010). Moreover, the influence of visceral fat accumulation and the presence of insulin resistance, may favor its development through inflammatory markers, such as interleukin-6 (IL-6) and tumor necrosis factor alpha (TNF-alpha) and the reduced concentrations of adiponectin, an important anti-inflammatory adipokine. This metabolic condition causes a higher lipase activity by increasing the influx of free fatty acids into the portal circulation, which are potentially hepatotoxic (Lam and Younossi, 2010; Ayonrinde et al, 2011).

Another contributing factor in the pathogenesis of NAFLD is the dietary pattern, rather than the high calorie food, the quality of the diet appears to play a key role in the development and progression of the disease. Diets high in saturated fat, cholesterol, and low in polyunsaturated fats, fibers and antioxidant vitamins C and E have been associated with this disease (Musso et al. 2003). Many studies investigated the association between NAFLD and carotid artery disease; below in the Table 2 are showed some results of different investigations.

Table 2. Investigations results of the association between NAFLD and the development of carotid artery disease

Author and year of publication	N sample	Study Design	Results
Moon SH et al. (2014)	755 healthy adult males who underwent a general health screening program.	Cross-sectional	Carotid F-fluorodeoxyglucose (FDG) positron emission tomography uptake, represented as maximum target-to-background ratio, was increased with mild (n= 237; 1.61 + 0.14; p= .033) and moderate NAFLD (n=145; 1.63 + 0.16; p=.005) compared with controls (n=373; 1.58 + 0.15). In patients aged >50 years, NAFLD was the only independent risk factor for high carotid FDG uptake (odds ratio, 2.12; 95% confidence interval, 1.10-4.07; p=.001).
Sanches PL et al. (2014)	79 obese adolescents were divided into two groups: 33 NAFLD and 46 non-NAFLD	Longitudinal	NAFLD is associated with cardiovascular risk factors and inflammatory markers of atherosclerosis that were positively correlated with cIMT only in the NAFLD group. Nevertheless, the strength of the present study is that the interdisciplinary therapy effectively improved cIMT and other proinflammatory adipokines in both groups.
Sinn DH et al. (2014)	10,581 consecutive male participants aged 30 years or older	Cross-sectional	2280 men diagnosed with fatty liver, and the mean age was 51.8 years old. Among them, 1797 were modest alcohol drinkers. The prevalence of carotid plaques (55.3% vs. 43.4%, p < 0.001) and carotid artery stenosis (11.0% vs. 5.5%, p < 0.001) was higher in non-drinkers than modest drinkers. Modest alcohol consumption had the independent inverse association with carotid plaques [odd ratio (OR): 0.74, 95% confidence interval (CI): 0.60-0.92] and carotid artery stenosis (OR: 0.62, 95% CI: 0.43-0.90), adjusted for age, smoking and metabolic syndrome.
Pacifico L et al. (2014)	548 children (aged 6–16 years), of whom 157 were normal-weight, 118 overweight, and 273 obese. Subjects were stratified into tertiles of TG/HDL-C.	Cross-sectional	The odds ratios for central obesity, insulin resistance, high hsCRP, NAFLD, metabolic syndrome, and elevated cIMT increased significantly with the increasing tertile of TG/HDL-C ratio, after adjustment for age, gender, pubertal status, and BMI-SDS. In a stepwise multivariate logistic regression analysis, increased cIMT was associated with high TG/HDL-C ratio [OR, 1.81 (95% CI, 1.08–3.04); p < 0.05], elevated BP [5.13 (95% CI, 1.03–15.08); p < 0.05], insulin resistance [2.16 (95% CI, 1.30–3.39); p < 0.01], and NAFLD [2.70 (95% CI, 1.62–4.56); p < 0.01].

Table 2. (Continued)

Author and year of publication	N sample	Study Design	Results
Kang JH et al. (2012)	320 non-diabetic patients with ultrasonographically diagnosed NAFLD and 313 non-diabetic patients without NAFLD who have less than 40 g alcohol/week drinking history.	Cross-sectional	NAFLD patients had a significantly increased mean carotid IMT (0.79 ± 0.18 vs. 0.73 ± 0.13 mm; $p < 0.001$) than those without the condition. The prevalence of increased IMT, defined as IMT ≥ 1 mm, and carotid plaque were 52.5% and 34.1% in the patients with NAFLD vs. 35.8% and 18.8% in the patients without this condition ($p < 0.001$). NAFLD-associated adjusted odds ratio for increased IMT was 1.236 [95% confidence interval (CI), 1.023-1.467, $p = 0.016$] without MetS and 1.178 (95% CI, 1.059-1.311, $p = 0.003$) with MetS. NAFLD-associated adjusted odds ratio of carotid plaque was 1.583 (95% CI, 1.309-1.857, $p = 0.024$) without MetS and 1.536 (95% CI, 0.512-4.604, $p = 0.444$) with MetS.
Caserta CA et al. (2010)	642 randomly selected adolescents aged 11-13 years	Cross-sectional	In univariate analysis, increased IMT was positively associated with the presence of NAFLD, body mass index (BMI), waist circumference, systolic blood pressure (all P's < 0.001), diastolic blood pressure ($P = 0.006$), gamma-glutamyl transpeptidase ($P = 0.006$), alanine aminotransferase ($P = 0.007$), and C-reactive protein ($P = 0.008$) and was inversely associated with high density lipoprotein cholesterol ($P < 0.001$).
Aygun C et al. (2008)	40 biopsy-proven NAFLD patients and 40 age-matched healthy control subjects	Case-control	The mean IMT was significantly higher in NAFLD patients (0.646 +/- 0.091 mm) than control subjects (0.544 +/- 0.067 mm), ($P < 0.001$).

NAFLD: non-alchoolic fatty liver disease; FDG: F-fluorodeoxyglucose; cIMT: carotid intima media thickness; CI: confidence interval; TG: triglycerides; HDL-C: high density lipoprotein-cholesterol; MeTS: metabolic syndrome; BMI: body mass index; IMT: intima media thickness.

Table 3. Criteria diagnose of Metabolic Syndrome

	OMS (1998)	NCEP-AT P III (2001)	IDF (2006)	IDF (2007) 6 to ≤ 10 years	IDF (2007) 10 to ≤ 16 years
Metabolic Syndrome diagnoses	Insulin Resistance + 2 components	3 of 5 components	Altered waist circumference + 2 components	-	Altered waist circumference + 2 components
COMPONENTS					
Insulin Resistance	IGT, IFG, DM type 2 or reduction in insulin sensibility	-	-	MetS cannot be diagnosed	-
Body Composition	Waist-hip ratio: Men: > 0,90 cm Women: > 0,85 cm and/or BMI > 30 kg/m²	Abdominal circumference: Men ≥ 102 cm Women ≥ 88 cm	Abdominal circumference: Men ≥ 94 cm Women ≥ 80 cm	Family factors that should be investigated by: - metabolic syndrome; - diabetes mellitus type II - dyslipidemia - cardiovascular disease - arterial hypertension - obesity	Waist circumference ≥ percentile 90 (according gender, age and ethnicity)
Serum Lipids (mg/dL)	Triglicerídeos ≥ 150 e/ou Homens HDL < 35 Mulheres HDL < 39	Triglicerídeos ≥ 150 e/ou Homens HDL < 40 Mulheres HDL < 50	Triglicerídeos ≥ 150 e/ou Homens HDL < 40 Mulheres HDL < 50 ou uso de hipolipemiantes		Triglycerides ≥ 150 HDL cholesterol< 40
Pressão Arterial (mmHg)	≥ 140/90	≥ 130/85 ou uso de anti-hipertensivos	≥ 130/85 ou uso de anti-hipertensivos		Sistolic ≥ 130 mmHg Diastolic ≥ 85 mmHg
Serum Glucose (mg/dL)	IGT, IFG or Diabetes Mellitus type 2	> 110 (including Diabetes Mellitus)	> 110 (including Diabetes Mellitus)	Waist circumference ≥ percentile 90 (according gender, age and ethnicity)	≥ 100 mg/dL or diabetes type 2
Others	Microalbuminúria Urinary albumin excretion≥ 20 µg/min	-	-		-

OMS: World Health Organization, NCEP-ATP III : National Cholesterol Education Program – Adult Treatment Panel III, IDF: International Diabetes Federation, DM: Diabetes mellitus, HDL: high density lipoprotein, IFG: Impaired fasting glucose; IGT: Impaired glucose tolerance, BMI: body mass index, MeTS: Metabolic Syndrome.

Table 4. Investigations results of the associations between Metabolic Syndrome and the development of Carotid Artery Disease

Author and year of publication	N sample	Study Design	Results
Wang ZH et al. (2012)	400 Chinese subjects were recruited, divided into control (n = 200) and MetS (n = 200) groups	Cross-sectional	The metabolic syndrome group showed significantly increased mean intima-media thickness (IMT (mean)) and significantly impaired carotid elastic properties (all P < 0.05), as compared to control group. Waist circumference (WC) was positively correlated with IMT (mean) (r = 0.130, P = 0.038), systolic carotid diameter (r = 0.139, P = 0.026) and diastolic carotid diameter (r = 0.168, P = 0.007). systolic blood pressure (SBP) and diastolic blood pressure were positively correlated with IMT(mean) (r = 0.201, P = 0.004; r = 0.168, P = 0.008, respectively).
Della-Morte D et al. (2010)	1133 Northern Manhattan Study subjects (mean age 65 +/- 9 years; 61% women; 58% Hispanic, 22% Black and 20% Caucasian).	Cross-sectional	The mean LogSTIFF (carotid artery stiffness) was 2.01 +/- 0.61 among those with the metabolic syndrome and 1.90 +/- 0.59 among those without the metabolic syndrome (P=0.003). The metabolic syndrome was significantly associated with increased logSTIFF in the final adjusted model (parameter estimate beta=0.100, P=0.01).
Toledo-Corral CM et al. (2009)	Ninety-seven healthy male and female overweight Latino children (mean age at baseline: 11.0+/-1.8 years)	Longitudinal	Persistent of metabolic syndrome over a 3-year period was associated with significantly higher carotid intima media thickness (0.647+/-0.018mm compared to 0.600+/-0.007mm in those who never had metabolic syndrome, p<0.01).

IMT: mean intima media thickness; WC: waist circumference; SBP: systolic blood pressure; STIFF: carotid artery stiffness; MetS: metabolic syndrome.

Metabolic Syndrome

The term metabolic syndrome was previously described as a clinical disease by Reaven in 1988 (Reaven, 1988). It was initially defined as a set of changes made by the presence of hyperinsulinemia, impaired glucose tolerance, low level of high density lipoprotein - cholesterol (HLD - cholesterol) and high triglyceride levels. Since then, this constellation of changes that comprise the metabolic syndrome has been updated by various organizations. Initially the definition was established by the World Health Organization in 1998, which the parameters of body mass index (BMI) were included, insulin resistance, microalbuminuria, hypertension as risk factors (Table 3) (Alberti and Zimmet, 1998).

In 2002 the definition criteria for metabolic syndrome was established by the National Cholesterol Education Program Adult Treatment Panel III (NCEP-ATP III). In 2005 a new diagnosis criteria was established by the International Diabetes Federation (IDF-2005) that was updated in 2007 including specific criteria for children and adolescents ($\leq$16 years) (Table 3) (Alberti et al. 2005; Alberti et al. 2007). Many metabolic complications that are presented in metabolic syndrome such as, increased waist circumference, insulin resistance and alterations in lipid profile are associated with the development and progression of carotid artery disease, suggesting the close relationship between metabolic syndrome and carotid artery dysfunction. It is demonstrated some investigations about this conception in Table 4.

Dyslipidemia

In obesity increased cardiovascular risk occurs by the interaction of factors associated with dyslipidemia, elevated blood glucose, insulin resistance and high blood pressure (Klop et al., 2013). Dyslipidemia state is closely linked to the presence of central obesity or the accumulation of visceral fat and is manifested by elevated total cholesterol (TC), elevated low-density lipoprotein (LDL), reduced high density lipoprotein (HDL) and elevated triglycerides (TG). Such changes may be related to excessive intake of fats and carbohydrates in the diet, genetic factors, use of certain medications and, in addition, other associated pathology, such as obesity (Howard et al., 2003).

All lipid content found in the blood is originated from two distinct forms by diet (corresponds to about 30%) or the endogenous production (70%). Triglycerides (TG) stemmed from food are transported via chylomicrons.

The formation of endogenous lipids occurs initially with the production of molecules of VLDL (very low-density lipoprotein) that originates in the liver by the clustering of lipids mainly TG. VLDL molecules are converted to intermediate density lipoproteins by lipoprotein lipase (LPL), may be captured again by the liver and undergo degradation of its components or action suffering form of hepatic lipase and lipoprotein LDL. On the other hand, the HDL lipoprotein that is produced by the liver and intestine, has the main function of reversing the cholesterol transport, a fundamental process for lipid homeostasis in peripheral cells. In addition to this, HDL cholesterol plays an important role to protect against the development of the atherogenic process promoting the removal of lipids oxidized LDL and inhibiting the attachment of adhesion molecules and monocytes to the vascular endothelium (Sanches and Dâmaso, 2012). In the Table 5, it is observed some investigations of the relationship between dyslipidemia and carotid artery complications.

Table 5. Investigations results of the association between Dyslipidemia and the development of Carotid Artery Disease

Author and year of publication	N sample	Study Design	Results
Fujihara K et al. (2013)	One hundred one Japanese patients	Cross-sectional	Male sex (p=0.031), systolic blood pressure (SBP) (p=0.039), and the LDL/HDL ratio (LDL/HDL) (p=0.013) were independent predictors of coronary artery stenosis and the LDL/HDL (p=0.042) independently predicted vulnerable coronary plaque by logistic regression analyses.
Chien KL et al. (2012)	2572 adults (mean age 53.8 years, 54.6% women)	Cross-sectional	Greater baseline LDL and blood pressure were associated with an increase in IMT (0.005 ± 0.002 mm per 1 mg/dL [p = 0.006] and 0.041 ± 0.004 mmHg [p <0.0001], respectively. Change in blood pressure was associated with a significant increase in IMT (0.047 ± 0.016, P = 0.004)
Magyar MT et al. (2004)	Eighty-six patients younger than 55 years	Cross-sectional	Intima-media thickness was larger in patient groups with high cholesterol levels than in the control group. Multiple regression model, IMT correlated positively with total cholesterol level (beta = 0.343; P = .002).

LDL: low-density lipoprotein, HDL: high lipoprotein density, IMT: intima media thickness; SBP: systolic blood pressure.

Diabetes

Diabetes mellitus is a condition characterized by a set of metabolic changes associated with hyperglycemia, resulting from changes in insulin secretion and insulin action which is the hormone that allows entry and utilization of glucose by tissues and organs (Oliveira and Moura, 2012).

The diagnosis of diabetes is based on the identification of hyperglycemia. Those used in diagnostic evaluations include assessment of random blood glucose, fasting blood glucose, glucose tolerance with a 75g in two hours test (GTT) and, in some cases, glycated hemoglobin (HbA1c) (WHO, 2006). Patients who exhibit the classic symptoms of hyperglycemia can be diagnosed when the plasma glucose value of 200 mg / dL or higher is found in a blood collection performed at any time (Oliveira and Moura, 2012) (Table 6).

Table 6. Possible Glucose Alterations during indetification of Diabetes Mellitus

Factors	Fasting glucose	Glucose Tolerance Test 2 hours after 75g of glucose	Casual glucose	Glycated Hemoglobin
Normal glucose	<110	<140	<200	-
Altered glucose	>110 e <126	-	-	-
Reduction in glucose tolerance	-	≥140 e <200	-	-
Diabetes Mellitus	<126	≥200	200	>6,5%

Fasting glucose: fasting regarded as no caloric intake for at least eight hours; Causal glycemia: defined as one that can be performed at any time of day without the presence of interval since the last meal; *Adapted from: Diabetes Brazilian Society (2009); World Health Organization (2006).*

Diabetes mellitus can be divided into two types: diabetes mellitus type 1 (DM1) and type 2 (DM2). The diabetes mellitus type 1 (DM1) accounts for only 5-10% of all cases of diabetes. It is also known as insulin-dependent diabetes mellitus, or juvenile diabetes, because it occurs most commonly in childhood and adolescence. However, diabetes mellitus type 2 (DM2) accounts for over 90% of diabetes cases, unlike DM1, DM2 is also known as insulin-independent, is commonly present in adults and exhibit obesity diagnosis or at least a buildup fat in the abdominal region (Kaul and Sharma, 2011). In the Table 7 it is possible to observe some studies that investigated the association between diabetes mellitus and the development of carotid artery disease.

Table 7. Investigations results of the association between Diabetes and the development of Carotid Artery Disease

Author and year of publication	N sample	Study Design	Results
Jae SY et al. (2012)	746 (age 53 ± 7 yrs) men with type 2 diabetes	Cross-sectional	Cardiorespiratory fitness was independently associated with common carotid intima media thickness in multivariable regression (β = -0.15, P < .05). After adjusting for established risk factors, high and moderate cardiorespiratory fitness were associated with lower odds ratios for having carotid atherosclerosis--0.49 (95% CI, 0.30-0.81), and 0.59 (95% CI, 0.38-0.92), respectively-- as compared with low cardiorespiratory fitness.
Polak JF et al. (2011)	1,116 participants (52% men) in the Epidemiology of Diabetes Interventions and Complications (EDIC) trial	Longitudinal	Albuminuria, older age, male sex, smoking, and higher systolic blood pressure were significant predictors of IMT progression.
Gómez-Marcos MA et al. (2011)	366 patients (105 diabetics and 261-non-diabetics)	Case serie-reports	Pulse wave velocity (PWV), ambulatory arterial stiffness index (AASI) and common carotid artery (CCA-IMT) were found to be greater in diabetic patients. CCA-IMT was independently correlated to the three measures of arterial stiffness in both groups. It was found increase in CCA-IMT of 0.40, 0.24 and 0.36 mm in diabetics, and of 0.48, 0.17 and 0.55 mm in non-diabetics. The variability of CCA-IMT was explained mainly by AASI, AIx and gender in diabetic patients, and by age, gender, AASI and PWV in non-diabetic patients.

IMT: intima media thickness, PWV: Pulse wave velocity, AASI: ambulatory arterial stiffness index, CCA: common carotid artery; CI: confidence interval.

Obesity and Carotid Artery Disease

Atherosclerosis is a chronic progressive disease, affecting the vascular wall of the arteries, such as carotid, and is characterized by the progressive accumulation of lipids and inflammatory cells within the intima of arteries. Carotid Intima media thickness (cIMT) is considered an important method of estimating precoce subclinical signal of atherosclerosis process. An increase of carotid artery is a result from endothelial dysfunction that creates lipid deposits in the intima of systemic arteries. The etiology of atherosclerosis is multifactorial, however the inflammation, metabolic alterations and endothelial dysfunction play pivotal role in this process (Schulz and Massber, 2014).

In this way, the carotid artery disease presents a close relation with obesity, which results from the link from visceral fat, inflammation and metabolic alterations commonly observed in obese individuals. Insulin resistance and inflammatory profile are described as risk factors related to increase values of carotid intima media thickness in obese adolescents. The exposure during childhood to these metabolic alterations may contribute to the development of atherosclerosis (de Lima Sanches et al., 2011, Sanches et al., 2012, Masquio et al., 2013) (Figure 3).

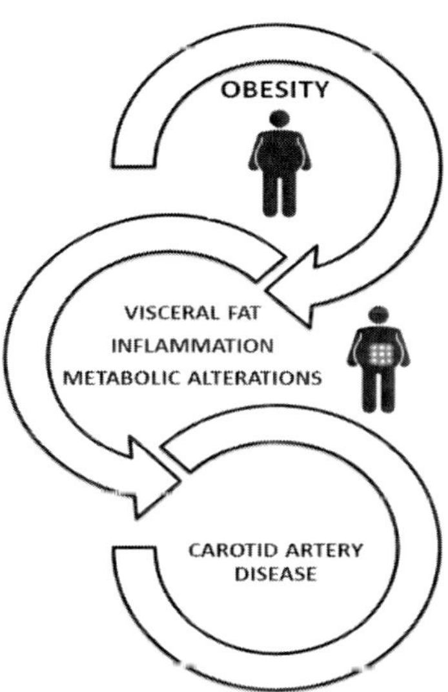

Figure 3. The link between obesity and carotid artery disease.

The normal artery contains three layers. The inner layer, the tunica intima, is lined by a monolayer of endothelial cells that is in contact with blood. The middle layer, or tunica media, contains smooth muscle cells embedded in a complex extracellular matrix. The adventitia, the outer layer of artery, contains mast cells, nerve endings and microvessels. The direct contact of endothelial cells with the blood flow means that they are particularly vulnerable to damage molecules in the blood on one hand, and that they have ideally "guard" roles on the other hand (Tang et al., 2014).

The atherosclerosis is characterized as a chronic inflammatory process that is initiated by alterations in metabolic parameters and together with endothelial cell dysfunction lead to the sub endothelial retention of low-density lipoproteins (LDL). This vascular lipid deposition in turn alerts the immune system. Consecutive local congregation of both adaptive and innate immune cells is a key step in atherogenesis, orchestrating the formation and progression of lipid-rich lesions or plaques (Schulz et al., 2014).

Endothelium dysfunction results from some risk factors, such as, hypertension, dyslipidemia and insulin resistance, which increase intima permeability to LDL molecules. The LDL cholesterol remains in the sub endothelial space, where they are oxidized (oxLDL) and stimulate expression of adhesion molecules, such as, Intercellular Adhesion Molecule 1 (ICAM-1) and Vascular Cell Adhesion Molecule 1 (VCAM-1), which act as an attraction for the early accession of serum leukocytes to endothelial cells. ICAM-1 and VCAM-1 are expressed on endothelial cells and mediate the adhesion and migration of leukocytes to the vascular endothelium, and thus might initiate inflammatory processes that eventually culminate in atherosclerotic lesions. Thus, ICAM-1 and VCAM-1 are considered as early markers of endothelial dysfunction and atherosclerosis. The mechanism that explains the expression of adhesion molecules by endothelial cells is partially mediated by increased expression of factor nuclear kappa B (NFkB), which activates the modified lipoproteins (oxLDL) and some inflammatory cytokines, such as, tumor necrosis factor alpha (TNF-α) and interleukin 6 (Sanches et al., 2009, Raederstorff et al., 2013).

The monocyte chemotactic proteins (MCP 1) induce migration of monocytes into the subendothelial space and their installation in the intima of arteries, where they take morphological characteristics of macrophages and increase the expression of scavenger receptors. These receptors are able to capture and internalize modified lipoproteins, such as oxLDL, and subsequently undergo a series of changes, resulting in the formation of foam cells. The macrophages located within the atheroma also secrete growing factors and cytokines, which are involved in the progression and complications of atherosclerosis (Sanches et al., 2009). Figure 4 illustrates the initial process of atherosclerosis.

Table 8. The role of adipokines and cytokines on atherosclerosis

Adipokines	Effects on atherosclerotic process
Adiponectin	Reduction of ICAM-1 and VCAM-1 expression
	Inhibition of monocytes adhesion to the endothelium
	Reduction in scavenger receptors expression
	Increase nitric oxide synthesis
	Inhibition of cytokine secretion by macrophages
	Inhibition of foam cell formation
TNF-α	Activation of NFkB
	Stimulation of migration and conversion of monocytes to macrophages
	Stimulation of IL-6 secretion
	Stimulation of endothelial cell apoptosis
	Reduction in endothelial-depending wall vasodilatation
CRP	Increase VCAM-1 and ICAM-1
	Increase monocytes recruitment in the endothelial wall
Interleukin 6	Increase VCAM-1, ICAM-1, interleukin 1 and MCP-1
	Increase hepatic secretion of CRP
	Increase fatty free acid influx
Leptin	Increase MCP 1 secretion by endothelial
	Stimulation of smooth muscle cells migration, proliferation and hypertrophy
	Stimulation of wall cells calcification
	Increase risks of thrombosis
PAI-1	Increase platelets and fibrin deposition in atheroma plaques
	Increases rupture of unstable atherosclerotic plaques and thrombus formation
Resistin	Increase VCAM-1 and ICAM-1
	Increase cytokines, MCP-1 and endotelin 1 production
	Stimulation of foam cell formation
	Increase TNF-a secretion by macrophages

ICAM-1: Intercellular Adhesion Molecule 1; VCAM-1: vascular cell adhesion molecule 1; NF-α: **tumor** necrosis factor alpha; IL-6: interleukin-6; CRP: C-reactive protein; MCP 1: monocyte chemotactic protein 1. *Adapted from Sanches et al., 2009*

The major clinical manifestations of atherosclerosis are coronary artery disease, leading to acute myocardial infarction (MI) and sudden cardiac death;

cerebrovascular disease, leading to stroke; and peripheral arterial disease, leading to ischemic limbs and viscera. These complications of atherosclerosis are leading causes of death worldwide (Mulder et al., 2014). In obese individual, both the increased secretion of adipokines by adipose tissue and cytokines secreted by macrophages participate of the atherogenesis process. Table 8 summarizes the main role of each adipokines/cytokine in this process.

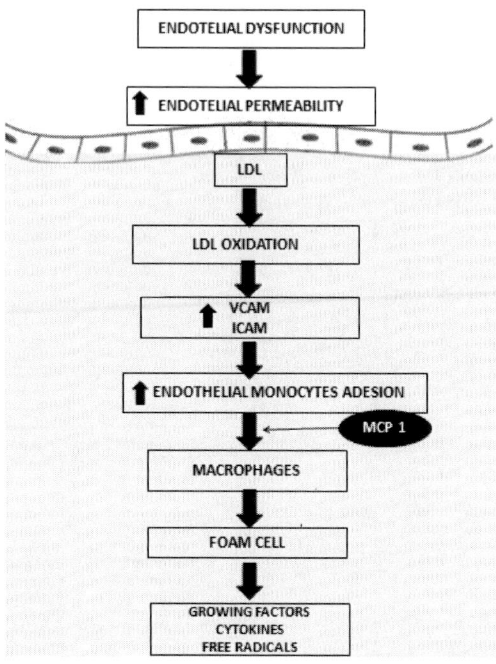

Figure 4. Atherosclerosis development.

Effects of Nutrition and Physical Exercise on Carotid Artery Disease

Nowadays it is well established the deleterious effects in the combination of inadequate diet and low physical exercise level in all population independent of age, gender and social class. The most commonly consequences of inadequate lifestyle is the increase in body mass, suggesting a development of obesity and consequently many comorbidities, including cardiovascular complications, in especially, carotid artery disease. Carotid artery disease also indicates patients at increased risk for fatal and nonfatal myocardial infarction. In the Cardiovascular Health Study, the 6-year risk for myocardial infarction or stroke was increased 3.6-fold to w40/1000 person-years in patients in the highest quintile of carotid intima-media thickness (IMT) (O'Leary et al., 1999).

Atherosclerosis can begin in relatively young individuals and continue to develop for many decades before clinical signs are observed or cardiovascular events occur. The first subclinical sign of atherosclerosis is an increase in arterial intima-media thickness (IMT), the result of endothelial dysfunction that leaves lipid deposits in the intima of systemic arteries (Järvisalo et al., 2001). Many hypotheses link obesity, endothelial dysfunction and subclinical signs of atherosclerosis in obese subjects (Sanches et al., 2010).

In obese adolescents, insulin resistance, visceral fat, leptin/adiponectin ratio and PAI-1 concentration were positive associated with carotid intima media thickness (cIMT). However, interdisciplinary weight loss treatment including nutritional, psychological, physiotherapy, clinical approach and physical exercise was effective in reducing these cardiovascular risk factors, including carotid intima media thickness and ICAM (Corgosinho et al., 2012, Sanches et al, 2012).

Accumulating evidence has demonstrated that structured physical exercise programs or even moderate levels of physical activity suppress cardiovascular morbidity and mortality in the whole population. Physical activity has been related inversely to the extent of atherosclerosis and the primary incidence of cardiovascular events (Belardinelli et al., 2001, Stampfer et al., 2000).

Interesting, in the review study of Kadoglou et al. (2008) the authors investigated the association of physical exercise with others therapies in carotid atherosclerosis in different kinds of study, including cross-sectional, observational and longitudinal interventions studies. Briefly the main findings showed in the investigation are presented in the table 9 below.

Furthermore, it was demonstrated that only more than 10.9 kg or 12.10% of weight loss was effective in reducing cIMT in obese adolescents. Moreover, weight loss was an independent predictor of controlling cIMT independently of age and gender (Masquio et al., 2013). Additionally, dietary patterns are widely recognized as contributors to cardiovascular and cerebrovascular disease. In this way, the diet can also influence carotid artery in obese patients.

Table 9. Effects of physical exercise in carotid artery

Author and year of publication	N sample	Study Design	Results
Sanches et al. (2012)	66 post-pubescent obese adolescents	Longitudinal The sample was were divided in two groups according to homeostasis model assessment of insulin resistance (HOMA-IR) measurement and submitted an interdisciplinary weight loss therapy	Simple linear regression analyze revealed ∆Visceral to be an independent predictor to reduction of cIMT in this group (R2 adjusted = 0.14, p = 0.04). The presence of insulin resistance can impair changes in cIMT leading to early development of atherosclerosis in obese adolescents submitted to an interdisciplinary intervention
Meyer AA et al. (2006)	67 obese subjects (14.7 +/- 2.2 years)	Longitudinal The effect of a 6-month exercise program in obese children on flow-mediated vasodilation (FMD) carotid intima-media thickness (IMT) and cardiovascular risk factors (CRF)	Reduce progression of maximum common carotid artery and carotid bifurcation intima-media thickness in the exercise group
Hägg U et al (2005)	29 healthy young male and female	Cross-sectional	Cardiovascular function (VO$_2$max) was inversely associated with intima-media thickness of common carotid artery measurement
Nordstrom CK et al (2003)	500 individuals	Observational Self-reported physical exercise time	Intima-media thickness declined from 14.3 +/- 1.7 microns per year in sedentary subjects, to 10.2 +/- 1.0 microns per year in moderately active subjects, to 5.5 +/- 1.5 microns per year in vigorously active subjects (p <0.0001)
Luedemann J et al. (2002)	1632 individuals aged 45 to 70 years	Cross-sectional Physical activity, dietary patterns, and cardiovascular risk factors were assessed in interviews with the use of standardized scales.	Significant decreasing trends were found for both intima-media thickness and severe asymptomatic atherosclerosis from unfavorable to optimal lifestyle patterns in never smokers but not in smokers. Regression analysis revealed an increased risk of severe asymptomatic atherosclerosis in subjects with an unfavorable lifestyle pattern compared with those with an optimal pattern (odds ratio 2.68; 95% CI, 1.13 to 6.37)

Author and year of publication	N sample	Study Design	Results
Okada K et al. (2004)	1390 male and female residents of a suburban Japanese town	Prospective study	After 2 years of follow-up, both sexes of both treatment groups showed significant reductions of TC, low-density lipoprotein cholesterol (LDL-C). Lifestyle modification can reduce carotid IMT in the general population, with or without the use of lipid-lowering drugs

HOMA-IR: homeostasis model assessment of insulin resistance; cIMT: carotid intima media thickness; FMD: flow-mediated vasodilation; CRF: cardiovascular risk factors; TC: total cholesterol; LDL-C: low-density lipoprotein-cholesterol.

Saturated Fatty Acid

Saturated fatty acids can predict cIMT. Confirming this, Bemelmans et al. (2002) demonstrated that cIMT was predicted by changes in saturated fatty intake estimated by food frequency questionnaire. In addition, a cross-sectional analyses conducted by Merchant et al. (2008) demonstrated that every 10g/day increase in saturated fatty intake was associated with increase of 0.03 mm on cIMT.

Recent evidence from our research group indicated that saturated fatty may potentiate inflammation, insulin resistance and metabolic syndrome parameters in obese adolescents, which are directly associated to atherosclerosis progression (Estadella et al., 2013, Masquio et al., 2014).

Moreover, the consumption of saturated fatty was correlated with LDL-cholesterol, an important risk factor related to atherosclerosis development. In adolescents, diet containing less saturated fatty acids contributes to a more beneficial lipid profile, which can contribute in avoiding atherosclerosis and LDL oxidation (Monge-Rojas et al., 2005, Breda et al., 2013).

Trans Fatty Acid

Recently, there has been continuing accumulation of evidence that trans fatty acid has potential harmful action in blood lipid metabolism, atherosclerosis development and cardiovascular disease (Dalainas and Ioannou, 2008).

There are two main sources of dietary trans fatty acids: those that occur naturally in meat and dairy products and those formed during the partial hydrogenation of vegetable fat. In their unmodified state, vegetable fats are made up of fatty acids with only cis double bonds. Traditionally, fats have been partially hydrogenated to increase their viscosity (changing vegetable fats from a liquid to a semi-liquid or solid) and/or extend their shelf life (decreasing susceptibility to oxidation). The major source of trans fatty acids in the food supply has come from foods made with partially hydrogenated fat, such as, found in many baked goods, snack foods, fast foods, margarines, and shortening, primarily commercially prepared fried and baked products. Dietary trans double bond containing fatty acids have been associated with increased risk of cardiovascular disease (Lichtenstein, 2014).

Trans fatty acid pattern habits were associated with higher cardiovascular risk, primarily attributable to higher risk of stroke in older adults. Trans fatty acid pattern was positively associated with progression of atherosclerosis (Imamura et al., 2012). In agreement, Merchant et al. (2008) demonstrated that 1-g/d higher intake of trans fat was associated with a 0.03-mm higher IMT in adult individuals after multivariate adjustment.

Furthermore, trans fatty can contribute to alteration in plasma lipids and insulin resistance, which can potentiate atherosclerosis process (Vermunt et al., 2001, Angelieri et al., 2012). In young adults, the high trans acid diet significantly increased the plasma LDL-:HDL-cholesterol ratio by 8.1% and the total cholesterol: HDL-cholesterol ratio by 5.1% compared with the low-trans diet. This was largely explained by an increase in LDL-cholesterol on the high-trans diet, while no change was observed in the low-trans group (Vermunt et al., 2001).

One Brazilian study demonstrated that the mean trans fatty acid intake was 5.0 g/day, accounting for 2.4% of total energy and 6.8% of total lipids. The adolescents had the highest mean intake levels (7.4 g/day; 2.9% of energy) while the adults and the elderly had similar intake (2.2% of energy for both; 6.4% of lipids and 6.5% of lipids, respectively). These results arise preoccupation, since trans fatty acid intake is above the level recommended by the World Health Organization, and can contribute to cardiovascular risks (Castro et al., 2009).

Antioxidants

Oxidative stress consists of unbalanced higher cellular levels of reactive oxygen species (ROS), which can lead to damage in cellular structures, like protein, DNA and lipid membranes, and can oxidize LDL to form atherogenic oxided LDL. Indeed, the oxidative stress has a key role in atherosclerosis development (Seifried et al., 2007; Kovacic, 2008).

Antioxidant capacity is considered by the ability to scavenge free oxygen and nitrogen species, abrogating the pro-inflammatory activity of ROS-generating enzymes such as cyclooxygenase (COX), lipoxygenase (LOX), and inducible nitric oxide synthase (iNOS) (Tangney and Rasmussen, 2013). Moreover, antioxidants may prevent atherosclerosis by interfering with endothelial activation, which involves the expression of endothelial adhesion molecules (Gianetti et al., 2002).

Vitamin C is an important component of the antioxidant system, and it has been suggested to reverse endothelial dysfunction in the coronary or peripheral arteries of patients with overt atherosclerosis or in those with conditions that predispose to atherosclerosis. In this way, Odermarsky et al. (2009) demonstrated that carotid artery intima-media thickness was higher in children and adolescents in the lowest tertile of vitamin C blood concentration than in those in the highest tertile.

Polyphenols are a group of chemical substances, characterized by the presence of more than one phenolic group whereas the phenolic acids are phenols with only one ring. Polyphenols belong to one of the major classes of plant secondary metabolites including, flavonoids, lignans, stilbenes, coumarins and tannins. Regular consumption of foods and beverages rich in polyphenols is associated with a reduction in the risk of a range of pathological conditions, ranging from hypertension to coronary heart disease and stroke (Ghosh and Scheepens, 2009).

Polyphenols may lower the risk of cardiovascular disease and chronic diseases due to their antioxidant and anti-inflammatory properties, as well as their beneficial effects on blood pressure, lipids and insulin resistance. Polyphenols modulate inflammation, lipid metabolism, improve antioxidant status and endothelial function, increase NO release, and protect against platelet aggregation. In agreement, among high-risk subjects, those who reported a high polyphenol intake, especially of stilbenes and lignans, showed a reduced risk of overall mortality compared to those with lower intakes (Tresserra-Rimbau et al., 2014). In obese individuals, diets naturally rich in polyphenols can reduce oxidative stress (Annuzzi et al., 2014).

The polyphenol resveratrol is found notably in grapes and in a variety of medicinal plants. Recently, resveratrol has been suggested to have cardioprotective effects (Raederstorff et al., 2013). Resveratrol has antithrombotic effects that appear to be the result of reduced susceptibility to platelet activation and aggregation, reduced synthesis of prothrombotic mediators (eicosainoid synthesis) and decreased gene expression of tissue factor. Indeed, resveratrol can inhibit platelet aggregation, activate eNOS and /or inhibit the generation of reactive oxygen species (Vilahur and Badimon, 2013)

Furthermore, it was shown that resveratrol inhibited ICAM-1 and VCAM-1 expression in endothelial cells through inhibition of nuclear factor-B (NF-kB) activation. Resveratrol at low dose (0.1 µmol/L) significantly inhibited the adhesion of monocytes to stimulated endothelial cells, a key step in the development of atherosclerosis (Raederstorff et al., 2013).

Agarwal et al. (2013) demonstrated that the expression of ICAM, VCAM, and IL-8 was significantly decreased in human coronary endothelial artery cells incubated with plasma from subjects who were supplemented with 400 mg/day resveratrol (and quercetin and grape skin extract) for 30 days. Resveratrol can also reduce serum MCP-1 and pro-inflammatory cytokine secretion (IL-6 and TNF-α) through downregulation of the NF-κB pathway as well as promote adiponectin expression and release from human adipose tissue (Tangney and Rasmussen, 2013).

Recently, meta-analyses of controlled trials concluded that endothelial function can be significantly improved in healthy adults in the initial 2 hour after intake of grape polyphenols. The acute effect of grape polyphenols on endothelial function may be more significant but the peak effect is delayed in subjects with a smoking history or coronary heart disease as compared with the healthy subjects (Li et al., 2013).

Dietary supplementation with pomegranate juice (which contains potent tannins and anthocyanins) during 4 years resulted in significant reduction of IMT after 1 year. The serum LDL basal oxidative state and LDL susceptibility to copper ion-induced oxidation were both significantly reduced, by 90% and 59%, respectively, after 12 months of pomegranate juice consumption. Furthermore, serum levels of antibodies against oxidized LDL were decreased by 19%. Systolic blood pressure was reduced after 1 year of pomegranate juice consumption by 12%. For all studied parameters, the maximal effects were observed after 1 year of supplementation (Aviram et al., 2004).

Olive oil is the common main component of the Mediterranean food pattern. A high consumption of olive oil (i.e. the highest quintile, with a median intake of 54.3 g/day) has been found associated with protection from myocardial infarction. Moreover, dietary olive oil was found to protect from total mortality in those who reported often or regularly consumption as compared with those reporting lower consumption (never or sometimes). Possible mechanistic explanations of this negative association of olive oil intake and cardiovascular diseases may be explained by the improvement of endothelial function or an anti-inflammatory activity on the vessel wall. Moreover, higher dietary consumption of olive oil was associated with lower values of carotid IMT in adults (Buil-Cosiales et al., 2008).

Conclusion and Future Direction

The development of carotid artery disease could be associated it many factors especially with metabolic alterations present in obesity. The pro-inflammatory state including hyperleptinemia framework, increase in interleukin-6, tumor necrosis factor-α, resistin, visfatin, apelin, plasminogen activator inhibitor-1 and reduction in adiponectin appears to be an interesting metabolic complications that contributing to the development of carotid artery diseases. In addition in the present chapter it was showed the association between obesity, comorbidities and cardiovascular risk factors such as non-alcoholic fatty liver disease, diabetes, metabolic syndrome and dyslipidemia. Finally, non pharmacological strategies as practice of physical exercise and healthy food intake seems to be important interventions associated with others therapies that could reduce and prevent cardiovascular risk factors.

References

Adams LA and Angulo P. Treatment of non-alcoholic fatty liver disease. *Postgraduate Medical Journal.* 2006; 82: 315–22.

Adams LA, Lymp JF, St Sauver J, Sanderson SO, Lindor KD, Feldstein A, Angulo P. The natural history of nonalcoholic fatty liver disease: a population-based cohort study. *Gastroenterology.* 2005; 129:113-21.

Agarwal B, Campen MJ, Channell MM, Wherry SJ, Varamini B, Davis JG, Baur JA, Smoliga JM. Resveratrol for primary prevention of atherosclerosis: clinical trial evidence for improved gene expression in vascular endothelium. *Int. J. Cardiol.* 2013; 166: 246-8.

Alberti KG, Zimmet P, Shaw J, IDF Epidemiology Task Force Consensus Group. The metabolic syndrome-a new world-wide definition. *Lancet* 2005; 366:1059-62.

Alberti KG, Zimmet P, Shaw J, IDF Epidemiology Task Force Consensus Group. The metabolic syndrome in children and adolescents. *Lancet* 2007; 369: 2059-61.

Alberti KG, Zimmet PZ: Definition, diagnosis and classification of diabetes mellitus and its complications. 1. Diagnosis and classification of diabetes mellitus provisional report of a WHO consultation. *Diabet Med.* 1998; 15: 539–53.

Angelieri CT, Barros CR, Siqueira-Catania A, Ferreira SR. Trans fatty acid intake is associated with insulin sensitivity but independently of inflammation. *Braz. J. Med. Biol. Res.* 2012; 45(7): 625-31.

Annuzzi G, Bozzetto L, Costabile G, Giacco R, Mangione A, Anniballi G, Vitale M, Vetrani C, Cipriano P, Della Corte G, Pasanisi F, Riccardi G, Rivellese AA. Diets naturally rich in polyphenols improve fasting and postprandial dyslipidemia and reduce oxidative stress: a randomized controlled trial. *Am. J. Clin. Nutr.* 2014; 99(3): 463-71.

Aviram M, Rosenblat M, Gaitini D, Nitecki S, Hoffman A, Dornfeld L, Volkova N, Presser D, Attias J, Liker H, Hayek T. Pomegranate juice consumption for 3 years by patients with carotid artery stenosis reduces common carotid intima-media thickness, blood pressure and LDL oxidation. *Clin. Nutr.* 2004; 23(3): 423-33.

Aygun C, Kocaman O, Sahin T, Uraz S, Eminler AT, Celebi A, Senturk O, Hulagu S. Evaluation of metabolic syndrome frequency and carotid artery intima-media thickness as risk factors for atherosclerosis in patients with nonalcoholic fatty liver disease. *Dig. Dis. Sci.* 2008; 53(5): 1352-7.

Ayonrinde OT, Olynyk JK, Beilin LJ, Mori TA, Pennell CE, de Klerk N, Oddy WH, Shipman P, Adams LA. Gender-specific differences in adipose distribution and adipocytokines influence adolescent nonalcoholic fatty liver disease. *Hepatology.* 2011; 53: 800-9.

Belardinelli R, Paolini I, Cianci G, Piva R, Georgiou D, Purcaro A. Exercise training intervention after coronary angioplasty: the ETICA trial. *J. Am. Coll Cardiol.* 2001; 37(7): 1891-900.

Bemelmans WJ, Lefrandt JD, Feskens EJ, Broer J, Tervaert JW, May JF, et al. Change in saturated fat intake is associated with progression of carotid and femoral intima-media thickness, and with levels of soluble intercellular adhesion molecule-1. *Atherosclerosis.* 2002; 163(1): 113-20.

Breda L, Di Marzio D, Giannini C, Gaspari S, Nozzi M, Scarinci A, Chiarelli F, Mohn A. Relationship between inflammatory markers, oxidant-antioxidant status and intima-media thickness in prepubertal children with juvenile idiopathic arthritis. *Clin. Res. Cardiol.* 2013; 102(1): 63-71.

Bruun JM, Pedersen SB, Kristensen K, Richelsen B. Effects of pro-inflammatory cytokines and chemokines on leptin production in human adipose tissue in vitro. *Mol. Cell Endocrinol.* 2002; 190(1-2): 91-9.

Buil-Cosiales P, Irimia P, Berrade N, Garcia-Arellano A, Riverol M, Murie-Fernández M, Martínez-Vila E, Martínez-González MA, Serrano-Martínez M. Carotid intima-media thickness is inversely associated with olive oil consumption. *Atherosclerosis.* 2008; 196(2): 742-8.

Caserta CA, Pendino GM, Amante A, Vacalebre C, Fiorillo MT, Surace P, Messineo A, Surace M, Alicante S, Cotichini R, Zuin M, Rosmini F, Mele A, Marcucci F. Cardiovascular risk factors, nonalcoholic fatty liver disease, and carotid artery intima-media thickness in an adolescent population in southern Italy. *Am. J. Epidemiol.* 2010; 171(11): 1195-202.

Castro MA, Barros RR, Bueno MB, César CL, Fisberg RM. Trans fatty acid intake among the population of the city of São Paulo, Brazil. *Rev Saude Publica.* 2009; 43(6): 991-7.

Cawthorn WP, Sethi JK. TNF-alpha and adipocyte biology. *FEBS Lett.* 2008; 582(1): 117-31.

Chien KL, Tu YK, Hsu HC, Su TC, Lin HJ, Chen MF, Lee YT. Differential effects of the changes of LDL cholesterol and systolic blood pressure on the risk of carotid artery atherosclerosis. *BMC Cardiovasc. Disord.* 2012; 12: 66.

Coppari R, Bjorbæk C. Leptin revisited: its mechanism of action and potential for treating diabetes. *Nat. Rev. Drug Discov.* 2012; 11(9): 692-708.

Corgosinho FC, de Piano A, Sanches PL, Campos RM, Silva PL, Carnier J, Oyama LM, Tock L, Tufik S, de Mello MT, Dâmaso AR. The role of PAI-1 and adiponectin on the inflammatory state and energy balance in obese adolescents with metabolic syndrome. *Inflammation.* 2012; 35(3): 944-51.

Dalainas I, Ioannou HP. The role of trans fatty acids in atherosclerosis, cardiovascular disease and infant development. *Int. Angiol.* 2008; 27(2): 146-56.

Dâmaso, AR; de Piano, A; Campos, RMS; Corgosinho, FC; Siegfried, W; Caranti, DA; Masquio, DCL; Carnier J; Sanches, PL; Silva, PL; Nascimento, CMO; Oyama, LM; Dantas, ADA; de Mello, MT; Tufik, S; Tock, L. Multidisciplinary Approach to Treat Obese Adolescents: Effects on Cardiovascular Risk Factors, Inflammatory Profile and Neuroendocrine Regulation of Energy Balance. *Int. J. Endocrinol.* 2013. doi:10.1155/2013/541032.

de Ferranti S, Mozaffarian D. The perfect storm: obesity, adipocyte dysfunction, and metabolic consequences. *Clin. Chem.* 2008; 54(6): 945-55.

de Lima Sanches P, de Mello MT, Elias N, Fonseca FA, de Piano A, Carnier J, Oyama LM, Tock L, Tufik S, Dâmaso AR. Improvement in HOMA-IR is an independent predictor of reduced carotid intima-media thickness in obese adolescents participating in an interdisciplinary weight-loss program. *Hypertens Res.* 2011; 34(2): 232-8.

DeBoer MD. Obesity, systemic inflammation, and increased risk for cardiovascular disease and diabetes among adolescents: a need for screening tools to target interventions. *Nutrition.* 2013; 29(2): 379-86.

Della-Morte D, Gardener H, Denaro F, Boden-Albala B, Elkind MS, Paik MC, Sacco RL, Rundek T. Metabolic syndrome increases carotid artery stiffness: the Northern Manhattan Study. *Int. J. Stroke.* 2010; 5(3): 138-44.

Dowman JK, Tomlinson JW, Newsome PN. Pathogenesis of non-alcoholic fatty liver disease. *QJM* 2010; 103: 71-83.

Egger G, Dixon J. Beyond Obesity and Lifestyle: A Review of 21st Century Chronic Disease Determinants. *Biomed. Res. Int.* 2014; 2014: 731685.

Eric A. Finkelstein, Justin G. Trogdon, Joel W. Cohen and William Dietz Annual Medical Spending Attributable To Obesity: Payer-And Service-Specific Estimates. *Health Affairs*, 28, no.5 (2009): w822-w831.

Estadella D, da Penha Oller do Nascimento CM, Oyama LM, Ribeiro EB, Dâmaso AR, de Piano A. Lipotoxicity: effects of dietary saturated and transfatty acids. *Mediators Inflamm.* 2013; 2013: 137579.

Fain JN, Madan AK, Hiler ML, Cheema P, Bahouth SW. Comparison of the release of adipokines by adipose tissue, adipose tissue matrix, and adipocytes from visceral and subcutaneous abdominal adipose tissues of obese humans. *Endocrinology.* 2004; 145(5): 2273-82.

Finucane MM, Stevens GA, Cowan MJ, Danaei G, Lin JK, Paciorek CJ, Singh GM, Gutierrez HR, Lu Y, Bahalim AN, Farzadfar F, Riley LM, Ezzati M; Global Burden of Metabolic Risk Factors of Chronic Diseases Collaborating Group (Body Mass Index). National, regional, and global trends in body-mass index since 1980: systematic analysis of health examination surveys and epidemiological studies with 960 country-years and 9·1 million participants. *Lancet.* 2011; 377(9765): 557-67.

Ford ES, Li C, Cook S, Choi HK. Serum concentrations of uric acid and the metabolic syndrome among US children and adolescents. *Circulation.* 2007; 115(19): 2526-32.

Fuentes E, Fuentes F, Vilahur G, Badimon L, Palomo I. Mechanisms of chronic state of inflammation as mediators that link obese adipose tissue and metabolic syndrome. *Mediators Inflamm.* 2013; 2013: 136584.

Fujihara K, Suzuki H, Sato A, Kodama S, Heianza Y, Saito K, Iwasaki H, Kobayashi K, Yatoh S, Takahashi A, Yamada N, Sone H, Shimano H. Carotid artery plaque and LDL-to-HDL cholesterol ratio predict atherosclerotic status in coronary arteries in asymptomatic patients with type 2 diabetes mellitus. *J. Atheroscler Thromb.* 2013; 20(5): 452-64.

Ghosh D, Scheepens A. Vascular action of polyphenols. *Mol. Nutr. Food Res.* 2009; 53(3): 322-31.

Gianetti J, Pedrinelli R, Petrucci R, Lazzerini G, De Caterina M, Bellomo G, De Caterina R. Inverse association between carotid intima-media thickness and the antioxidant lycopene in atherosclerosis. *Am. Heart J.* 2002; 143(3): 467-74.

Giordano A, Murano I, Mondini E, Perugini J, Smorlesi A, Severi I, Barazzoni R, Scherer PE, Cinti S. Obese adipocytes show ultrastructural features of stressed cells and die of pyroptosis. *J. Lipid Res.* 2013; 54(9): 2423-36.

Gómez-Marcos MA, Recio-Rodríguez JI, Patino-Alonso MC, Agudo-Conde C, Gómez-Sánchez L, Rodríguez-Sánchez E, Martín-Cantera C, García-Ortiz L. Relationship between intima-media thickness of the common carotid artery and arterial stiffness in subjects with and without type 2 diabetes: a case-series report. *Cardiovasc. Diabetol.* 2011; 10(1): 3.

Hägg U, Wandt B, Bergström G, Volkmann R, Gan LM. Physical exercise capacity is associated with coronary and peripheral vascular function in healthy young adults. *Am. J. Physiol. Heart Circ. Physiol.* 2005; 289(4): H1627-34.

Howard BV, Ruotolo G, Robbins DC. Obesity and dyslipidemia. *Endocrinol. Metab. Clin. North Am* 2003; 32: 855-67.

Imamura F, Lemaitre RN, King IB, Song X, Lichtenstein AH, Matthan NR, Herrington DM, Siscovick DS, Mozaffarian D. Novel circulating fatty acid patterns and risk of cardiovascular disease: the Cardiovascular Health Study. *Am. J. Clin. Nutr.* 2012; 96(6): 1252-61.

Instituto Brasileiro de Geografia e Estatística. POF 2008-2009 - Antropometria e estado nutricional de crianças, adolescentes e adultos no Brasil. 2010. Available on: http://www.ibge.gov.br/home/presidencia/noticias/noticia_visualiza.php?id_noticia=1699&id_pagina=1 Acessed on june 13, 2014.

Jae SY, Heffernan K, Fernhall B, Choi YH. Cardiorespiratory fitness and carotid artery intima media thickness in men with type 2 diabetes. *J. Phys. Act Health.* 2012; 9(4): 549-53.

Järvisalo MJ, Jartti L, Näntö-Salonen K, Irjala K, Rönnemaa T, Hartiala JJ, Celermajer DS, Raitakari OT. Increased aortic intima-media thickness: a marker of preclinical atherosclerosis in high-risk children. *Circulation.* 2001; 104(24): 2943-7.

Kadoglou NP, Iliadis F, Liapis CD. Exercise and carotid atherosclerosis. *Eur. J. Vasc. Endovasc. Surg.* 2008; 35(3): 264-72.

Kang JH, Cho KI, Kim SM, Lee JY, Kim JJ, Goo JJ, Kim KN, Jhi JH, Kim DJ, Lee HG, Kim TI. Relationship between Nonalcoholic Fatty Liver Disease and Carotid Artery Atherosclerosis Beyond Metabolic Disorders in Non-Diabetic Patients. *J. Cardiovasc. Ultrasound.* 2012; 20(3): 126-33.

Kaul A, Sharma J. Impact of bariatric surgery on comorbidities. *Surg Clin North Am.* 2011; 91: 1295-312.

Kelsey MM, Zaepfel A, Bjornstad P, Nadeau KJ. Age-related consequences of childhood obesity. *Gerontology.* 2014; 60(3): 222-8.

Klop B, Elte JW, Cabezas MC. Dyslipidemia in obesity: mechanisms and potential targets. *Nutrients.* 2013; 5: 1218-40.

Kovacic, P; Somanathan, R. Unifying mechanism for eye toxicity: electron transfer, reactive oxygen species, antioxidant benefits, cell signaling and cell membranes. *Cell Membr Free Radic. Res.* 2008; 2: 56-69.

Kralisch S, Klein J, Lossner U, Bluher M, Paschke R, Stumvoll M, Fasshauer M. Interleukin-6 is a negative regulator of visfatin gene expression in 3T3-L1 adipocytes. *Am. J. Physiol. Endocrinol. Metab.* 2005; 289(4): E586-90.

Kusminski CM, da Silva NF, Creely SJ, Fisher FM, Harte AL, Baker AR, Kumar S, McTernan PG. The in vitro effects of resistin on the innate immune signaling pathway in isolated human subcutaneous adipocytes. *J. Clin. Endocrinol. Metab.* 2007; 92(1): 270-6.

Lam B, Younossi ZM. Treatment options for nonalcoholic fatty liver disease. *Therap. Adv. Gastroenterol.* 2010; 3: 121-37.

Lavie CJ, McAuley PA, Church TS, Milani RV, Blair SN. Obesity and cardiovascular diseases: implications regarding fitness, fatness, and severity in the obesity paradox. *J. Am. Coll Cardiol.* 2014; 63(14): 1345-54.

Leal Vde O, Mafra D. Adipokines in obesity. *Clin. Chim. Acta.* 2013; 419: 87-94.

Lee S, Bacha F, Gungor N, Arslanian SA. Racial differences in adiponectin in youth: relationship to visceral fat and insulin sensitivity. *Diabetes Care.* 2006; 29(1): 51-6.

Li SH, Tian HB, Zhao HJ, Chen LH, Cui LQ. The acute effects of grape polyphenols supplementation on endothelial function in adults: meta-analyses of controlled trials. *PLoS One.* 2013; 8(7): e69818.

Lichtenstein AH. Dietary trans Fatty acids and cardiovascular disease risk: past and present. *Curr. Atheroscler Rep.* 2014; 16(8): 433.

Luedemann J, Schminke U, Berger K, Piek M, Willich SN, Döring A, John U, Kessler C. Association between behavior-dependent cardiovascular risk factors and asymptomatic carotid atherosclerosis in a general population. *Stroke.* 2002; 33(12): 2929-35.

Magyar MT, Paragh G, Katona E, Valikovics A, Seres I, Csiba L, Bereczki D. Serum cholesterols have a more important role than triglycerides in determining intima-media thickness of the common carotid artery in subjects younger than 55 years of age. *J. Ultrasound. Med.* 2004; 23(9): 1161-9.

Masquio DC, de Piano A, Campos RM, Sanches PL, Corgosinho FC, Carnier J, Oyama LM, do Nascimento CM, de Mello MT, Tufik S, Dâmaso AR. Saturated fatty acid intake can influence increase in plasminogen activator inhibitor-1 in obese adolescents. *Horm Metab Res.* 2014; 46(4): 245-51.

Masquio, DC; de Piano, A; Sanches, PL; Corgosinho, FC; Campos, RM; Carnier, J; da Silva, PL; Caranti, DA; Tock, L; Oyama, LM; Oller do Nascimento, CM; de Mello, MT; Tufik S; Dâmaso, AR. The effect of weight loss magnitude on pro-/anti-inflammatory adipokines and carotid intima-media thickness in obese adolescents engaged in interdisciplinary weight loss therapy. *Clin. Endocrinol* (Oxf). 2013; 79(1): 55-64.

Merchant AT, Kelemen LE, de Koning L, et al. Interrelation of saturated fat, trans fat, alcohol intake, and subclinical atherosclerosis. *Am. J. Clin. Nutr.* 2008; 87(1): 168-174.

Meyer AA, Kundt G, Lenschow U, Schuff-Werner P, Kienast W. Improvement of early vascular changes and cardiovascular risk factors in obese children after a six-month exercise program. *J. Am. Coll Cardiol.* 2006; 48(9): 1865-70.

Ministério da Saúde. Vigitel - Vigilância de Fatores de Risco e Proteção para Doenças Crônicas por Inquérito Telefônico. Available on: http://portalsaude.saude.gov.br/images/pdf/2014/abril/30/Lancamento-Vigitel-28-04-ok.pdf. Acessed june 13, 2014.

Monge-Rojas R, Campos H, Fernández Rojas X. Saturated and cis- and trans-unsaturated fatty acids intake in rural and urban Costa Rican adolescents. *J. Am. Coll Nutr.* 2005; 24(4): 286-93.

Moon SH, Noh TS, Cho YS, Hong SP, Hyun SH, Choi JY, Kim BT, Lee KH. Association Between Nonalcoholic Fatty Liver Disease and Carotid Artery Inflammation Evaluated by 18F-Fluorodeoxyglucose Positron Emission Tomography. *Angiology.* 2004; pii: 0003319714537872.

Mulder WJ, Jaffer FA, Fayad ZA, Nahrendorf M. Imaging and Nanomedicine in Inflammatory Atherosclerosis. *Sci. Transl. Med.* 2014; 6(239): 239sr1.

Musso G, Gambino R, De Michieli F, Cassader M, Rizzetto M, Durazzo M, Fagà E, Silli B, Pagano G. Dietary habits and their relations to insulin resistance and postprandial lipemia in nonalcoholic steatohepatitis. *Hepatology.* 2003; 37: 909-16.

Nordstrom CK, Dwyer KM, Merz CN, Shircore A, Dwyer JH. Leisure time physical activity and early atherosclerosis: the Los Angeles Atherosclerosis Study. *Am. J. Med.* 2003; 115(1): 19-25.

Odermarsky M, Lykkesfeldt J, Liuba P. Poor vitamin C status is associated with increased carotid intima-media thickness, decreased microvascular function, and delayed myocardial repolarization in young patients with type 1 diabetes. *Am. J. Clin. Nutr.* 2009; 90(2): 447-52.

Okada K, Maeda N, Tatsukawa M, Shimizu C, Sawayama Y, Hayashi J. The influence of lifestyle modification on carotid artery intima-media thickness in a suburban Japanese population. *Atherosclerosis.* 2004; 173(2): 329-37.

O'Leary DH, Polak JF, Kronmal RA, Manolio TA, Burke GL, Wolfson SK Jr. Carotid-artery intima and media thickness as a risk factor for myocardial infarction and stroke in older adults. Cardiovascular Health Study Collaborative Research Group. *N. Engl. J. Med.* 1999; 340(1): 14-22.

Oliveira CAM, Moura RF. Diabetes In: Dâmaso, A. Nutrição e Exercício Físico na Prevenção de Doenças, Guanabara Koogan: Rio de Janeiro. 2012; 142-60.

Pacifico L, Bonci E, Andreoli G, Romaggioli S, Di Miscio R, Lombardo CV, Chiesa C. Association of serum triglyceride-to-HDL cholesterol ratio with carotid artery intima-media thickness, insulin resistance and nonalcoholic fatty liver disease in children and adolescents. *Nutr. Metab. Cardiovasc. Dis.* 2014; 24(7): 737-43.

Piya MK, McTernan PG, Kumar S. Adipokine inflammation and insulin resistance: the role of glucose, lipids and endotoxin. *J. Endocrinol.* 2013; 216(1): T1-T15.

Polak JF, Backlund JY, Cleary PA, Harrington AP, O'Leary DH, Lachin JM, Nathan DM; DCCT/EDIC Research Group. Progression of carotid artery intima-media thickness during 12 years in the Diabetes Control and Complications Trial/Epidemiology of Diabetes Interventions and Complications (DCCT/EDIC) study. *Diabetes.* 2011; 60(2): 607-13.

Raederstorff D, Kunz I, Schwager J. Resveratrol, from experimental data to nutritional evidence: the emergence of a new food ingredient. *Ann. N Y Acad. Sci.* 2013; 1290: 136-41.

Reaven GM: Banting lecture 1988. Role of insulin resistance in human disease. *Diabetes* 1988; 37: 1595-1607.

Sanches Pde L, Mello MT, Fonseca FA, Elias N, Piano Ad, Carnier J, Tock L, Oyama LM, Tufik S, Dâmaso A. Insulin resistance can impair reduction on carotid intima-media thickness in obese adolescents. *Arq Bras. Cardiol.* 2012; 99(4): 892-8.

Sanches PL, Dâmaso A. Dislipidemias In: Dâmaso, A. Nutrição e Exercício Físico na Prevenção de Doenças, Guanabara Koogan: Rio de Janeiro. 2012; 97-108.

Sanches PL, Naccarato GAF, Xavier AD and Dâmaso AR. Obesidade e doença artério-coronariana. In: Dâmaso A. Obesidade. – 2 ed.- Rio de Janeiro: Guanabara Koogan, 2009.

Sanches, PL; de Mello, MT; Elias, N; Fonseca, FA; Campos, RM; Carnier, J; de Piano, A; Masquio, DC; Silva, PL; Oyama, LM; Corgosinho, FC; Nascimento, CM; Tock, L; D'Elia, CA; Tufik, S; Dämaso, AR. Hyperleptinemia: Implications on the Inflammatory State and Vascular Protection in Obese Adolescents Submitted to an Interdisciplinary Therapy. Inflammation, 2013

Sanches, PL; Mello, MT; Tock, L; Tufik, S; Oyama, LM; Dâmaso, A. The Influence of Insulin Resistance on Inflammatory and Subclinical Markers of Atherosclerosis in Obese Adolescents. *Arq. Bras. Cardiol.*, 2012, 56, 12-17.

Sanches PL, de Piano A, Campos RM, Carnier J, de Mello MT, Elias N, Fonseca FA, Masquio DC, da Silva PL, Corgosinho FC, Tock L, Oyama LM, Tufik S, Dâmaso AR. Association of nonalcoholic fatty liver disease with cardiovascular risk factors in obese adolescents: the role of interdisciplinary therapy. *J. Clin. Lipidol.* 2014; 8(3): 265-72.

Schulz C, Massberg S. Atherosclerosis-Multiple Pathways to Lesional Macrophages. *Sci. Transl. Med.* 2014; 6(239): 239ps2.

Seifried, HE; Anderson, DE; Fisher, EI; Milner, JA. A review of the interaction among dietary antioxidants and reactive oxygen species. *J. Nutr. Biochem.* 2007; 18: 567-579.

Sinn DH, Gwak GY, Cho J, Son HJ, Paik YH, Choi MS, Lee JH, Koh KC, Paik SW, Yoo BC. Modest alcohol consumption and carotid plaques or carotid artery stenosis in men with non-alcoholic fatty liver disease. *Atherosclerosis.* 2014; 234(2): 270-5.

Stampfer MJ, Hu FB, Manson JE, Rimm EB, Willett WC. Primary prevention of coronary heart disease in women through diet and lifestyle. *N. Engl. J. Med.* 2000; 343(1): 16-22.

Tang X, Luo YX, Chen HZ, Liu DP. Mitochondria, endothelial cell function, and vascular diseases. *Front Physiol.* 2014; 5: 175.

Tangney CC, Rasmussen HE. Polyphenols, inflammation, and cardiovascular disease. *Curr. Atheroscler Rep.* 2013; 15(5): 324.

Tilg H, Moschen AR. Inflammatory mechanisms in the regulation of insulin resistance. *Mol. Med.* 2008; 14(3-4): 222-31.

Tock L, Prado WL, Caranti DA, Cristofalo DM, Lederman H, Fisberg M, Siqueira KO, Stella SG, Antunes HK, Cintra IP, Tufik S, de Mello MT, Dâmaso AR. Nonalcoholic fatty liver disease decrease in obese adolescents after multidisciplinary therapy. *Eur. J. Gastroenterol. Hepatol.* 2006; 18(12): 1241-5.

Toledo-Corral CM, Ventura EE, Hodis HN, Weigensberg MJ, Lane CJ, Li Y, Goran MI. Persistence of the metabolic syndrome and its influence on carotid artery intima media thickness in overweight Latino children. *Atherosclerosis.* 2009; 206(2): 594-8.

Tresserra-Rimbau A, Rimm EB, Medina-Remón A, Martínez-González MA, López-Sabater MC, Covas MI, Corella D, Salas-Salvadó J, Gómez-Gracia E, Lapetra J, Arós F, Fiol M, Ros E, Serra-Majem L, Pintó X, Muñoz MA, Gea A, Ruiz-Gutiérrez V, Estruch R, Lamuela-Raventós RM; PREDIMED Study Investigators. Polyphenol intake and mortality risk: a re-analysis of the PREDIMED trial. *BMC Med.* 2014; 12(1): 77.

Vázquez-Vela ME, Torres N, Tovar AR. White adipose tissue as endocrine organ and its role in obesity. *Arch. Med. Res.* 2008; 39(8): 715-28.

Vermunt SH, Beaufrère B, Riemersma RA, Sébédio JL, Chardigny JM, Mensink RP; TransLinE Study. Dietary trans alpha-linolenic acid from deodorised rapeseed oil and plasma lipids and lipoproteins in healthy men: the TransLinE Study. *Br. J. Nutr.* 2001; 85(3): 387-92.

Vilahur G, Badimon L. Antiplatelet properties of natural products. *Vascul. Pharmacol.* 2013; 59(3-4): 67-75.

Wang ZH, Gong HP, Shang YY, Tang MX, Fang NN, Jiang GH, Zhang Y, Zhong M, Zhang W. An integrative view on the carotid artery alterations in metabolic syndrome. *Eur. J. Clin. Invest.* 2012; 42(5): 496-502.

World Health Organization. Obesity Situation and trends. http://www.who.int/gho/ncd/risk_factors/obesity_text/en/ Accessed June 10, 2014

World Health Organization. Available on: http://www.who.int/mediacentre/factsheets/fs311/en/ . Accessed June 10, 2014.

WHO. World Health Organization. Diet, Nutrition And The Prevention Of Chronic Diseases. 2003. http://whqlibdoc.who.int/trs/who_trs_916.pdf. Accessed June 10, 2014.

World Health Organization. Definition and diagnosis of diabetes mellitus and intermediate hyperglycemia : report of a WHO/IDF consultation. Geneva, 2006.

Yamauchi T, Kamon J, Waki H, Terauchi Y, Kubota N, Hara K, Mori Y, Ide T, Murakami K, Tsuboyama-Kasaoka N, Ezaki O, Akanuma Y, Gavrilova O, Vinson C, Reitman ML, Kagechika H, Shudo K, Yoda M, Nakano Y, Tobe K, Nagai R, Kimura S, Tomita M, Froguel P, Kadowaki T. The fat-derived hormone adiponectin reverses insulin resistance associated with both lipoatrophy and obesity. *Nat. Med.* 2001; 7(8): 941-6.

Zimmet P, Alberti G, Kaufman F, Tajima N, Silink M, Arslanian S, Wong G, Bennett P, Shaw J, Caprio S; International Diabetes Federation Task Force on Epidemiology and Prevention of Diabetes. The metabolic syndrome in children and adolescents. *Lancet.* 2007; 369(9579): 2059-61.

English Reviewed By:
Carolina Ackel D'Elia PhD.
Post Graduate Program of Nutrition, Universidade Federal de São Paulo - UNIFESP

Flávia Campos Corgosinho MSc.
Post Graduate Program of Nutrition, Universidade Federal de São Paulo - UNIFESP

In: Carotid Artery Disease
Editor: Sherri Derricks

ISBN: 978-1-63321-859-8
© 2014 Nova Science Publishers, Inc.

Chapter 5

Asymptomatic Carotid Disease: How Confident Are We About the Benefit of Endarterectomy?

George Ntaios, MD, MSc.[1]*,
Erietta Polychronopoulou, MD*[2]
and Konstantinos Makaritsis, MD, PhD[3]
[1](ESO Stroke Medicine), PhD, FESO,
Assistant Professor of Internal Medicine. Department of Medicine,
Larissa University Hospital,
School of Medicine, University of Thessaly, Larissa, Greece
[2]Department of Medicine, Larissa University Hospital, Larissa, Greece
[3]Assistant Professor of Internal Medicine, Department of Medicine,
Larissa University Hospital, School of Medicine,
University of Thessaly, Larissa, Greece

* Corresponding author: George Ntaios MD, MSc (ESO Stroke Medicine), PhD, FESO. Assistant Professor of Internal Medicine, Department of Medicine, Larissa University Hospital, School of Medicine, University of Thessaly. Biopolis 41110, Larissa, Greece. T; +30 241 3502888, F: +30 241 3501557, E-mail: gntaios@med.uth.gr.

Abstract

Currently, there is a wide discussion about the role of carotid endarterectomy in asymptomatic carotid disease. Current guidelines recommend that it is *"reasonable to perform carotid endarterectomy in asymptomatic patients with >70% internal carotid artery stenosis if the risk of perioperative stroke, myocardial infarction and death is low"*. This recommendation is largely based on two randomized controlled trials of carotid endarterectomy (CEA) which were performed more than a decade ago in patients with asymptomatic carotid stenosis. However, more recent data suggest that perhaps we cannot rely on these trials to guide our clinical practice nowadays. In this context, many scientists underline the need for new trials which are indeed ongoing. Moreover, nowadays there are several imaging techniques available which assist us to identify which carotid plaques are associated with the higher stroke risk.

Introduction

Carotid atheromatous disease is a common cause of ischaemic stroke [1] and the treatment of carotid artery stenosis has been a topic of intense debate over the last 30 years. Randomized trials have shown the efficacy of carotid endarterectomy in secondary stroke prevention while carotid stenting represents a less invasive alternative to surgical intervention. Advances in medical therapy have led to improvement in the outcome of atherosclerotic carotid stenosis. However, the optimal management of symptomatic and asymptomatic carotid disease remains still controversial. The benefits of surgical intervention in severe symptomatic stenosis have been well documented by the North American Symptomatic Carotid Endarterectomy Trial (NASCET) [2] and European Carotid Surgery Trial (ECST) [3] trials. Recently, there is emerging evidence in favor of aggressive medical management which may reduce the compelling indications for interventional treatment especially in asymptomatic patients.

A wide discussion is currently ongoing with regards to the effect of carotid endarterectomy in patients with asymptomatic carotid disease. Current guidelines from the American Heart Association/American Stroke Association recommend that it is *"reasonable to perform carotid endarterectomy in asymptomatic patients with >70% internal carotid artery stenosis if the risk of perioperative stroke, myocardial infarction and death is low"* [4].

Similar recommendation is available also from the European Society of Cardiology [5]. These recommendations are mainly guided by two randomized controlled trials of carotid endarterectomy (CEA) which were performed more than a decade ago in patients with asymptomatic carotid stenosis [6, 7]. However, subsequent studies indicate that perhaps these trials cannot be relied on to guide current clinical practice. Hence, new trials are currently ongoing to confirm the findings of the older studies. Additionally, several imaging techniques are available nowadays to aid in the identification of the carotid plaques which are associated with the higher stroke risk.

Randomized Controlled Trials of Carotid Endarterectomy in Asymptomatic Carotid Stenosis

The Asymptomatic Carotid Artery Stenosis (ACAS) trial was performed between 1987 and 1993 in 39 clinical sites and was published in the JAMA in 1995 [6]. It recruited 1662 patients aged between 40 and 79 years with unilaterally or bilaterally asymptomatic, hemodynamically significant carotid stenosis of 60% or greater reduction in diameter, who were randomized to carotid endarterectomy or not, on top of 325mg of aspirin daily plus the best medical treatment available at the period that the trial was performed. The definition of hemodynamically significant carotid stenosis required at least one of three criteria: arteriography within the previous two months showing a stenosis of >60% reduction in diameter, doppler examination within the previous two months showing a frequency or velocity greater than the instrument-specific threshold with 95% positive predictive value or Doppler examination within the previous two months showing a frequency or velocity greater than the instrument-specific 90% positive predictive value threshold confirmed by ocular pneumoplethysmographic [8]. After a median follow-up of 2.7 years and 4657 patient-years, the 5-years aggregate risk for ipsilateral stroke and any perioperative stroke or death was 5.1 % for surgical patients and 11.0% for patients treated medically (aggregate risk reduction of 53% [95% confidence interval, 22% to 72%]) [6].

The Asymptomatic Carotid Surgery Trial (ACST) was a multicenter randomized controlled trial which was performed between 1993 and 2003 in 126 clinical sites and was published in Lancet in 2004 [7]. It randomized approximately 3120 patients with asymptomatic carotid stenosis to immediate

CEA or indefinite deferral of any CEA. The follow-up was up to 5 years. The inclusion criteria included the presence of severe unilateral or bilateral carotid artery stenosis (reduction of >60% on ultrasound) which had not caused any stroke, transient cerebral ischaemia, or other relevant neurological symptoms in the past 6 months and that both the physician and patient were substantially uncertain whether to perform immediate CEA or deferral of any CEA until a more definite need. The 30-days stroke or death risk after CEA was 3.1% (95% CI 2.3–4.1). Patients who were randomized to immediate CEA had reduced 5-year stroke risk compared to patients allocated to referral (6.4% vs. 11.8%, i.e. a difference of 5.4% [95%CI 3.0–7.8], p<0·0001), and in particular for fatal or disabling strokes (3.5% vs. 6.1%, i.e. a difference of 2.5% [95%CI 0.8–4.3], p=0.004) and fatal strokes (difference of 2.1% [95%CI 0.6–3.6], p=0.006). The results were similar when perioperative events were excluded (3.8% vs. 11%, i.e. a difference of 7.2% [95%CI 5.0–9.4], p<0·0001). This effect was mainly due to carotid territory ischaemic strokes (2.7% vs 9.5%, i.e. a difference of 6.8% [95%CI 4.8–8.8], p<0·0001), and in particular disabling or fatal strokes (1.6% vs. 5.3%, i.e. a difference of 3.7% [95%CI 2.1–5.2], p<0·0001), as well as perioperative strokes. Benefit was significantly different between males and females, and between <65 and 65-74 years of age [7].

These two randomized controlled trials weighed heavily towards the 2011 guidelines of the American Heart Association and the American Stroke Association which suggested that *"it is reasonable to perform carotid endarterectomy in asymptomatic patients with >70% internal carotid artery stenosis if the risk of perioperative stroke, myocardial infarction and death is low"* [4].

Similarly, the European Stroke Cardiology guidelines, which are endorsed by the European Stroke Organization, recommend that *"in asymptomatic patients with carotid artery stenosis ≥60%, CEA should be considered as long as the perioperative stroke and death rate for procedures performed by the surgical team is <3% and the patient's life expectancy exceeds 5 years"* [5].

Best Medical Treatment: Then and Now

These two randomized controlled trials received significant criticism and many scientists raised serious concerns that they can't be relied on to guide our clinical practice nowadays. Several arguments have been highlightened: firstly, in the ACST trial, the number of patients needed to treat (NNT) to prevent one fatal stroke or perioperative death in five years was 40, which is considered by many experts as a relatively large number for such an aggressive, radical, etiological treatment like endarterectomy [9]. Secondly, the "best medical treatment" which was available at the period that the trials were performed can't be considered "best" nowadays, as outlined below [10].

Antiplatelets

The antiplatelet agent that most of the participants of these two trials received was acetylsalicylic acid. However, nowadays more antiplatelets choices are available which perhaps are more efficacious than acetylsalicylic acid: clopidogrel is an inhibitor of platelet aggregation induced by adenosine diphosphate. In 1996, the results of the CAPRIE trial were published. CAPRIE was a randomized, blinded, trial which assessed the efficacy and safety of clopidogrel (75 mg once daily) compared to aspirin (325 mg once daily) to reduce the risk of a composite outcome cluster of ischaemic stroke, myocardial infarction, or vascular death in patients with atherosclerotic vascular disease manifested as either recent ischaemic stroke, recent myocardial infarction, or symptomatic peripheral arterial disease. The follow-up ranged between 1 to 3 years with a mean value of 1.9 years. A total of 19185 patients were recruited in 384 clinical sites and 16 countries. There were 1960 first outcome events; on the intention-to treat analysis, patients on clopidogrel had an annual 5.3% risk of ischaemic stroke, myocardial infarction, or vascular death compared to 5.8% in the aspirin arm (i.e. a statistically significant relative-risk reduction of 8.7% in favor of clopidogrel (95%CI 0.3–16.5, p=0·043] without major differences in safety [11].

Another antiplatelet choice which is available nowadays is the combination of aspirin with dipyridamole. The ESPRIT was a randomised controlled open trial designed to determine the efficacy of this combination compared to aspirin for the secondary prevention of vascular events in patients with ischaemic stroke. In this study 2739 patients with a previous ischaemic stroke of arterial origin were randomized to 30-325mg aspirin daily or to the same dose of aspirin combined with 200mg of dipyridamole twice daily. The primary endpoint was the composite of vascular death, non-fatal stroke, non-fatal myocardial infarction, or major bleeding complication. The mean time of follow-up was 3.5 years and the median aspirin dose was 75 mg in both treatment groups (range 30-325mg). During the trial, 389 patients had at least one primary endpoint: 173 (13%) in the aspirin/dipyridamole arm versus 216

(16%) in the aspirin arm. The absolute risk reduction of 1.0% per year (95%CI: 0.1-1.8%) corresponds to a NNT of 104 per year for the combination regimen to prevent death from all vascular causes, non-fatal stroke, non-fatal myocardial infarction, or major bleeding complication compared to monotherapy. When the ESPRIT data were included in the meta-analysis of previous trials, there was an overall risk ratio for the composite of vascular death, stroke, or myocardial infarction of 0.82 (95%CI 0.74–0.91). It needs to be noticed that the ESPRIT trial was not blinded with regards to treatment allocation. However, all members of the auditing committee that classified the outcome events, were unaware of the allocated study treatment. Other limitations of the study included the long duration of the clinical trial (up to 8 years) and the non-standarized dose of aspirin. Also, the authors acknoledge that the classification of large or small vessel disease based on clinical features was not the ideal method, since about 10–20% of strokes that were classified as lacunar on the basis of clinical features actually represented a cortical infarct and vice versa. Ideally, the classification should be based on diffusion weighted MR, which was not routinely available for the patients of this trial [12].

Statins

The lipid-lowering treatment, and in particular statins, is another cornerstone of stroke prevention which was significantly implemented in clinical practice during the recent years but was only moderately implemented in the ACST and ACAS trials. In the ACST trial, approximately 30% of patients were not receiving statin during the study: for patients recruited between 1993 and 1996, only approximately 10-15% of patients were started on lipid-lowering treatment, with the numbers being only moderately increased in the later periods (approximately 30% and 60% in the 1997-1999 και 2000-2003 periods respectively). It is noteworthy that at the end of the trial, only approximately 70% of patients were on lipid-lowering treatment [7].

During the recent years, several studies proved the beneficial effect of statins on cardiovascular prevention and stroke prevention in particular. The Stroke Prevention by Aggressive Reduction in Cholesterol Levels (SPARCL) was a randomized controlled trial which aimed to investigate whether treatment with 80 mg of atorvastatin per day would reduce the risk of fatal or nonfatal stroke among patients with a history of stroke or TIA [13]. During the trial, 4731 patients who had had a stroke or TIA within one to six months before recruitment, low-density lipoprotein (LDL) cholesterol levels between 100 and 190 mg/dl and no previously diagnosed coronary heart disease were randomized to double-blind treatment with 80 mg of atorvastatin per day or placebo[13]. The mean LDL cholesterol level during the trial was 73 mg/dl in the atorvastatin arm and 129 mg/dl in the placebo arm. After a median follow-up of 4.9 years, 265 patients (11.2%) in the atorvastatin group and 311 patients (13.1%) in the placebo arm suffered a fatal or nonfatal stroke, which corresponds to a 5-year absolute risk reduction of 2.2% (adjusted hazard ratio: 0.84, 95% CI: 0.71-0.99, p=0.03). There were 218 ischemic strokes and 55 hemorrhagic strokes in the atorvastatin group, and 274 ischemic strokes and 33 hemorrhagic strokes in the placebo group. There was a 3.5% (hazard ratio: 0.80, 95%CI 0.69-0.92, p=0.002) 5-years absolute risk reduction of major cardiovascular events, whereas the overall mortality rate was similar (216 deaths in the atorvastatin group and 211 deaths in the placebo group, p=0.98), as well as the serious adverse events. It should be noticed that elevated liver enzyme values were more common in patients taking atorvastatin.

Several post-hoc analyses of the SPARCL trial were published which showed that the beneficial effect of atorvastatin is evident in all patient subgroups regardless of age, gender, presence of carotid disease and type of stroke, with the exception of intracranial hemorrhage as the entry event [14-16]. In particular, in a subgroup analysis of 1007 patients with documented carotid stenosis and 3271 without, there was no heterogeneity in the treatment effect for the primary (fatal and nonfatal stroke) and secondary end points between the group with and without carotid stenosis. Among patients with carotid stenosis, atorvastatin was associated with a 33% reduction in the risk of any stroke (hazard ratio 0.67, 95% CI 0.47-0.94, p=0.02), and a 43% reduction in risk of major coronary events (HR 0.57, 95%CI 0.32-1.00, p=0.05). Similarly, later carotid revascularization was reduced by 56% (HR 0.44, 95% CI 0.24-0.79, p=0.006) in the atorvastatin arm [17].

Another cornerstone trial was the JUPITER which was a randomized controlled trial with the aim to investigate the effect of rosuvastatin in primary prevention. In this trial, 17802 patients with elevated high sensitivity C-reactive protein (CRP>2.0mg/l) but without dyslipidemia (<130mg/dl) were randomized to 20mg rosuvastatin daily or placebo. The primary endpoint included myocardial infarction, stroke, arterial revascularization, hospitalization for unstable angina, or death from cardiovascular causes. The trial was prematurely terminated after a median follow-up of 1.9 years. Rosuvastatin decreased LDL cholesterol levels by 50% and high-sensitivity C reactive protein levels by 37% compared to placebo. Per 100 person-years of follow-up, there were 0.77 and 1.36 primary endpoints (hazard ratio for rosuvastatin 0.56, 95% CI: 0.46-0.69, p=0.00001), 0.17 and 0.37 myocardial infarctions (hazard ratio, 0.46, 95%CI, 0.30-0.70; p=0.0002), 0.18 and 0.34 strokes (hazard ratio 0.52, 95% CI 0.34-0.79, p=0.002), 0.41 and 0.77 revascularization procedures or cases of unstable angina (hazard ratio 0.53, 95% CI 0.40-0.70, p=0.00001), 0.45 and 0.85 combined end points of myocardial infarction, stroke, or death from cardiovascular causes (hazard ratio, 0.53, 95% CI 0.40-0.69, p=0.00001), and 1.00 and 1.25 deaths from any cause (hazard ratio 0.80, 95% CI 0.67-0.97, p=0.02) in the rosuvastatin and placebo groups respectively. There was no sign of heterogeneity in any of the subgroups evaluated. There were similar rates of myopathy or cancer in the two trial arms, but the rosuvastatin group had a higher rate of diabetes [18, 19].

The aforementioned evidence indicates that not only the antiplatelet arm, but also the lipid-lowering arm of the asymptomatic carotid endarterectomy trials were suboptimal according to current standards and definitely cannot be considered as best medical treatment nowadays. And indeed, this improvement in medical treatment during the recent years seems to be associated with a parallel improvement in patient outcome. As mentioned above, the percentage of the patients in the ACAS trial who were operated for carotid stenosis and suffered a stroke was 1.5 % during the follow-up. It is interesting to notice that later studies and published series of non-randomized patients with carotid stenosis who were not operated and received medical treatment only showed that the later the study is, the lower the risk for stroke is, with the trendline showing that nowadays the estimated risk of stroke for patients with carotid stenosis who are not operated is notably low and certainly much lower than the 1,5 % of the surgical arm of ACAS study [20]. These results confirm that the evolution of the medical treatment, notably of the antiplatelet and the lipid-lowering arms, affected positively and significantly the outcome of patients with carotid stenosis who receive only medical treatment and are not operated.

CEA Periprocedural Risk: Then and Now

It should be noticed that the low periprocedural risk reported in the aforementioned randomized controlled trials was not confirmed in subsequent real-world studies. In the ACAS trial, the periprocedural mortality risk was only 0.14%. However, in subsequent non-randomized studies in patients operated for carotid stenosis, the periprocedural mortality risk was much higher compared to the randomized trials [21]. The most plausible explanation for this finding lies in the strict inclusion and exclusion criteria of these trials to allow a surgeon to participate. In particular, in order for a surgeon to be accepted in the trial, he had to have an annual record of 12 endarterectomies with a mortality/morbidity rate of less than 3% [8]. As a result, 40% of the initial applicants were rejected [6]. But even for the surgeons who made it to the trial, if someone had two serious complications like stroke or death, he was temporarily excluded from the trial [8]. As a result, the surgeons that participated in these trials were highly selected and obviously were not representative of the general surgeon population that performs carotid endarterectomy procedures in daily clinical practice, thus possibly introducing selection bias in the trial.

So, how much can we rely on these trials nowadays to guide our clinical practice when, on one hand, the medical treatment has improved so much that perhaps overcomes the benefit of endarterectomy and, on the other hand, the safety profile of endarterectomy was not confirmed in the real-world setting? It is possible that perhaps we would not be able to reproduce the results of these trials if they were to be conducted again today. On the other hand, a recently published retrospective study showed that "optimal medical therapy" (OMT) did not prevent carotid disease progression or development of ipsilateral symptoms in almost half of patients with asymptomatic moderate carotid disease [22]; however, criticism was raised about this study that the OMT and non-OMT groups were not clearly distinguished and that current OMT was not accurately defined [23]. The aforementioned evidence clearly indicates the need for new trials of CEA in patients with carotid stenosis which will implement all aspects of up-to-date cardiovascular prevention. Indeed, as outlined below, there are already such trials ongoing.

Ongoing Trials of CEA in Asymptomatic Carotid Stenosis

There are two such trials currently ongoing: the SPACE-2 and the AMTEC trials. The AMTEC is a prospective randomized parallel, two-arm, multicenter trial with the aim to compare the efficacy of carotid endarterectomy along with best medical therapy versus best medical therapy alone in patients with asymptomatic extracranial carotid 70-79% stenosis. The screening study is performed with an ultrasound examination of all extracranial segments of brachiocephalic arteries. The field of interest is the atherosclerotic plaque at the bifurcation and the ostium of the common carotid artery and also the proximal segment of the internal carotid artery. The treatment plan includes lifestyle changes, smoking cessation consultation, and diabetes and obesity management for all patients. All participants receive antiplatelet therapy with aspirin at a dose 81-325mg daily and atorvastatin at a dose 10-80mg daily with a target of LDL<100mg/dl. In case that the LDL target is not achieved, patients receive extended release niacin, fibrates or ezetimibe. All patients receive also anti-hypertensive therapy with amlodipine (minimum 5mg) and losartan (minimum 50mg) with initial blood pressure target <130/80mmHg. In cases that this target is not reached, the dose is doubled and if still not enough, hydrochlorothiazide is added [24].

The SPACE-2 trial is a randomized, controlled, open, multicenter trial with three parallel groups: a) the best medical treatment (BMT) arm, b) the CEA in addition to BMT arm, and c) the CAS in addition to BMT arm. Patients are aged between 50 and 85 years, have a carotid stenosis of ≥70% and have no stroke or stroke-like symptoms due to the stenosis within the last 180 days. A hierarchical design is followed in an estimated population of 3640 patients in approximately 100 sites: firstly, a superiority trial of intervention (carotid artery stenting or carotid endarterectomy) vs. state-of-the-art medical-only treatment is performed. In case of superiority of the interventions, a noninferiority analysis will be tested between carotid artery stenting and carotid endarterectomy. All patients are treated with a regimen addressing individual patients' risk factor profile including lipid-lowering and antiplatelets. Patients are followed-up for up to 5 years. The primary safety endpoint is the rate of any stroke and overall-cause death within 30 days of treatment, whereas the primary efficacy end point is the cumulative rate of any stroke (i.e. ischaemic or haemorrhagic) or overall-cause death from any cause within 30 days plus an ipsilateral ischaemic stroke within 5 years of follow-up [25, 26].

How to Identify a High-Risk Carotid Plaque?

Until the results of these trials come available, it is doubtful whether a patient with an asymptomatic carotid stenosis should be operated. Perhaps, one approach could be to operate only those patients who are at high risk for future ipsilateral strokes, i.e. patients with a high-risk carotid atherosclerotic lesion. Imaging may have an important role in the selection of patients who may benefit from CEA given that nowadays there are several parameters which may be used to quantify the risk associated with an atherosclerotic carotid plaque.

Obviously, the degree of stenosis is one of the most important predictors of stroke risk associated with a carotid plaque. In an analysis of the severity of stenosis and plaque surface morphology assessed on the angiograms of the symptomatic carotid artery in 3007 patients in the European Carotid Surgery Trial[3], the degree of narrowing of the vessel lumen was still an independent predictor of ischemic stroke within 2 years of presentation [27].

Moreover, the plaque surface is another important predictor of stroke risk in patients with carotid atherosclerotic plaques. It seems that plaques with a regular surface are associated with lower stroke risk compared to plaques with irregular surface: in the same analysis from the European Carotid Surgery Trial, the angiographic plaque surface irregularity was associated with an increased risk of ipsilateral ischemic stroke on medical treatment for all degrees of stenosis ((hazard ratio 2.75, 95%CI: 1.30 to 5.80, p=0.01) [27].

Also, the total plaque area is also independently associated with stroke risk. An analysis in 6584 individuals from the Tromso population health study in 1994 to 1995 showed that the total plaque area appears to be a strong predictor for first-ever ischemic stroke [28]. The adjusted hazard ratio for 1 standard-deviation increase in square-root-transformed plaque area was 1.23 (95% CI 1.09–1.38, p=0.0009) in men and 1.19 (95%CI, 1.01–1.41, p=0.04) in women when adjusted for other cardiovascular risk factors. The multivariable-adjusted hazard ratio in the highest quartile of plaque area versus no plaque was 1.73 (95% CI, 1.19–2.52, p=0.004) in men and 1.62 (95% CI, 1.04–2.53, p=0.03) in women [28].

Furthermore, the fibrous cap was also associated with increased stroke risk, i.e. carotid plaques with thick fibrous cap are associated with lower stroke risk compared to plaques with thin or ruptured fibrous cap. In an analysis of 154 consecutive individuals with an initially asymptomatic 50% to 79% carotid stenosis, patients were followed clinically every three months. After a follow-up of 38.2 months, the Cox regression analysis identified a significant association between baseline MRI identification of a thin or ruptured fibrous cap and subsequent symptoms during follow-up (hazard ratio 17.0, p=0.001). In addition, other imaging parameters which were identified as additional independent predictors of outcome included intraplaque hemorrhage (hazard ratio 5.2, p=0.005), larger mean intraplaque hemorrhage area (IPH) (hazard ratio for 10mm^2 increase 2.6, p=0.006), larger maximum %lipid-rich/necrotic core (hazard ratio for 10% increase 1.6, p=0.004) and larger maximum wall thickness (hazard ratio for a 1mm increase 1.6, p=0.008) [29].

As mentioned in the aforementioned study, the presence of intraplaque hemorrhage in MRI constitutes a major marker of plaque instability. Singh et al. performed a retrospective analysis to investigate the association between magnetic resonance (MR) IPH in the carotid artery wall and the risk of subsequent ipsilateral cerebrovascular events in men with asymptomatic moderate carotid stenosis by using a rapid three-dimensional T1-weighted fat-suppressed spoiled gradient-echo sequence. They identified 91 men (mean age 74.8 years, range 47–88 years) who attended a vascular clinic between 2003 and 2006 with asymptomatic carotid stenosis (50%–70% at Doppler ultrasonography), who had undergone MR imaging for IPH detection: among them, 75 men with 98 eligible carotid arteries were included in the study and were followed for a minimum of 1 year (mean follow-up 24.9 months, range 12–43 months). Of the 98 carotid arteries that were included, 36 (36.7%) had an MR depicted IPH. Among carotids with IPH, there were six cerebrovascular events (two strokes and four transient ischemic attacks) compared to no clinical events in the carotid arteries without IPH. MR-depicted IPH was associated with a higher risk for cerebrovascular events (hazard ratio 3.59, 95%CI 2.48-4.71, p<0.001). Also, MR-depicted IPH negatively predicted outcomes with a negative predictive value of 100%. The results showed that MR-depicted IPH is associated with future ipsilateral cerebrovascular events whereas absence of an MR-depicted IPH is a reassuring marker of plaque stability and of a lower risk for future events [30]. Similar results were also shown in symptomatic patients with carotid artery disease in a prospective longitudinal cohort study of symptomatic patients with mild to moderate (30%-69%) carotid stenosis. Sixty-four patients were followed up for a median of 28 months (interquartile range 26-30) after imaging for IPH using MRI. Among them, 39 (61%) ipsilateral arteries showed intraplaque hemorrhage. Five ipsilateral strokes and 14 ipsilateral ischemic events occurred during the follow-up. Thirteen of these ischemic events, of which five were strokes, occurred in those with ipsilateral carotid intraplaque hemorrhage (hazard ratio 9.8, 95%CI 1.3-75.1) confirming that MR IPH is a reliable predictor of ipsilateral stroke and TIA in patients with symptomatic mild to moderate (30%-69%) carotid stenosis [31].

In addition, the ACES trial provided valuable information about the role of microembolic detection during transcranial Doppler (TCD) for the estimation of stroke risk in patients with asymptomatic carotid disease [32]. In this prospective observational study in patients with asymptomatic carotid stenosis of at least 70%, 467 patients from 26 centers worldwide had two 1-hour TCD recordings from the ipsilateral middle cerebral artery at baseline and one 1 h recording at 6, 12, and 18 months aiming to detect microembolic signals. Patients were followed up for 2 years and the primary outcome was ipsilateral stroke and transient ischaemic attack. Embolic signals were identified in 77 of 467 patients at baseline. The hazard ratio for the risk of ipsilateral stroke and transient ischaemic attack from baseline to 2 years in patients with embolic signals compared with those without embolic signals was 2.54 (95%CI 1.20–5.36, p=0.015), whereas for ipsilateral stroke alone, it was 5.57 (95%CI 1.61–19.32, p=0.007). Similarly, the absolute annual risk of ipsilateral stroke or transient ischaemic attack between baseline and 2 years was 7.13% in patients with embolic signals and 3.04% in patients without embolic signals. The hazard ratio for ipsilateral stroke was 3.62% in patients with embolic signals and 0.70% in patients without embolic signals. These results clearly indicate that detection of asymptomatic embolization on TCD can be a useful tool to evaluate the risk for stroke and transient ischaemic attack of a patient with asymptomatic carotid stenosis: patients with microembolic signals have higher risk for stroke or transient ischaemic attack compared to patients without microembolic signals) [32]. These results were also confirmed by a meta-analysis of studies of the association of embolic signals with future risk of ipsilateral stroke or ipsilateral stroke or transient ischaemic attack which showed that in 1144 patients, the hazard ratio for the risk of ipsilateral stroke for those with embolic signals compared with those without was 6.63 (95%CI 2.85–15.44, p<0·0001) without any heterogeneity between studies (p=0·33). Similarly, the hazard ratio for the risk of ipsilateral stroke and TIA for those with embolic signals compared with those without was 7.57 (95%CI 2.32–24.69; p=0·0008) with some heterogeneity between included studies (p=0·002) [32-37]. Moreover, similar conclusions were also drawn from patients with symptomatic carotid disease where microembolic signals were shown to predict stroke risk [38, 39].

More evidence came out recently from a retrospective analysis from the deferred endarterectomy arm of the Asymptomatic Carotid Surgery Trial (ACST) [40]. In this analysis, patients were followed up for ≥5 years with serial carotid duplex examinations, and data were derived from information obtained at randomization and annual follow-up visits with carotid duplex examination. Among 1469 patients included in the analysis, 244 (17%) had ipsilateral events, 240 had ipsilateral carotid surgery; 370 died from non-stroke causes and 82 had an asymptomatic carotid occlusion. The annual incidence of progression in the cohort as a whole was 5.2%. Of interest, diabetes and previous contralateral symptoms showed a significant independent association with ipsilateral neurological events. Ipsilateral events were associated with increased rates of progression over 1 year but not with low progression rates or regression. Hence, the clinical implication of this analysis is that fast rates of progression of carotid narrowing should be interpreted as a marker of significantly increased risk of future ipsilateral events. Also, duplex measurements showing a slow rate of progression of an asymptomatic carotid stenosis over 1 year should not be interpreted as a sign of increased risk of future events [40].

So, in conclusion, there are several good data showing that perhaps we cannot rely on the endarterectomy trials which were performed twenty years ago to guide our clinical practice nowadays, and we need new trials which are actually being performed. Moreover, we now have several imaging techniques to assist us identify the patients who are in high stroke risk and probably have the higher potential to benefit from endarterectomy.

References

[1]   Michel P, Odier C, Rutgers M, Reichhart M, Maeder P, Meuli R, et al. The Acute STroke Registry and Analysis of Lausanne (ASTRAL): design and baseline analysis of an ischemic stroke registry including acute multimodal imaging. *Stroke; a journal of cerebral circulation.* 2010;41:2491-8.

[2]   North American Symptomatic Carotid Endarterectomy Trial C. Beneficial effect of carotid endarterectomy in symptomatic patients with high-grade carotid stenosis. *The New England journal of medicine.* 1991;325:445-53.

[3]   Randomised trial of endarterectomy for recently symptomatic carotid stenosis: final results of the MRC European Carotid Surgery Trial (ECST). *Lancet.* 1998;351:1379-87.

[4]   Brott TG, Halperin JL, Abbara S, Bacharach JM, Barr JD, Bush RL, et al. 2011 ASA/ACCF/AHA/AANN/AANS/ACR/ASNR/CNS/SAIP/ SCAI/SIR/SNIS/SVM/SVS guideline on the management of patients with extracranial carotid and vertebral artery disease. *Stroke; a journal of cerebral circulation.* 2011;42:e464-540.

[5] European Stroke O, Tendera M, Aboyans V, Bartelink ML, Baumgartner I, Clement D, et al. ESC Guidelines on the diagnosis and treatment of peripheral artery diseases: Document covering atherosclerotic disease of extracranial carotid and vertebral, mesenteric, renal, upper and lower extremity arteries: the Task Force on the Diagnosis and Treatment of Peripheral Artery Diseases of the European Society of Cardiology (ESC). *European heart journal.* 2011;32:2851-906.

[6] Endarterectomy for asymptomatic carotid artery stenosis. Executive Committee for the Asymptomatic Carotid Atherosclerosis Study. *JAMA: the journal of the American Medical Association.* 1995;273:1421-8.

[7] Halliday A, Mansfield A, Marro J, Peto C, Peto R, Potter J, et al. Prevention of disabling and fatal strokes by successful carotid endarterectomy in patients without recent neurological symptoms: randomised controlled trial. *Lancet.* 2004;363:1491-502.

[8] Study design for randomized prospective trial of carotid endarterectomy for asymptomatic atherosclerosis. The Asymptomatic Carotid Atherosclerosis Study Group. *Stroke; a journal of cerebral circulation.* 1989;20:844-9.

[9] Chaturvedi S. Should the multicenter carotid endarterectomy trials be repeated? *Archives of neurology.* 2003;60:774-5.

[10] Sillesen H. What does 'best medical therapy' really mean? European journal of vascular and endovascular surgery : *the official journal of the European Society for Vascular Surgery.* 2008;35:139-44.

[11] Committee CS. A randomised, blinded, trial of clopidogrel versus aspirin in patients at risk of ischaemic events (CAPRIE). CAPRIE Steering Committee. *Lancet.* 1996;348:1329-39.

[12] Group ES, Halkes PH, van Gijn J, Kappelle LJ, Koudstaal PJ, Algra A. Aspirin plus dipyridamole versus aspirin alone after cerebral ischaemia of arterial origin (ESPRIT): randomised controlled trial. *Lancet.* 2006;367:1665-73.

[13] Amarenco P, Bogousslavsky J, Callahan A, 3rd, Goldstein LB, Hennerici M, Rudolph AE, et al. High-dose atorvastatin after stroke or transient ischemic attack. *The New England journal of medicine.* 2006;355:549-59.

[14] Huisa DN, Stemer AB, Zivin JA. Atorvastatin in stroke: a review of SPARCL and subgroup analysis. *Vascular health and risk management.* 2010;6:229-36.

[15]	Amarenco P, Benavente O, Goldstein LB, Callahan A, 3rd, Sillesen H, Hennerici MG, et al. Results of the Stroke Prevention by Aggressive Reduction in Cholesterol Levels (SPARCL) trial by stroke subtypes. *Stroke; a journal of cerebral circulation.* 2009;40:1405-9.

[16]	Chaturvedi S, Zivin J, Breazna A, Amarenco P, Callahan A, Goldstein LB, et al. Effect of atorvastatin in elderly patients with a recent stroke or transient ischemic attack. *Neurology.* 2009;72:688-94.

[17]	Sillesen H, Amarenco P, Hennerici MG, Callahan A, Goldstein LB, Zivin J, et al. Atorvastatin reduces the risk of cardiovascular events in patients with carotid atherosclerosis: a secondary analysis of the Stroke Prevention by Aggressive Reduction in Cholesterol Levels (SPARCL) trial. *Stroke; a journal of cerebral circulation.* 2008;39:3297-302.

[18]	Scheen AJ. [JUPITER: reduction by rosuvastatin of cardiovascular events and mortality in healthy subjects without hyperlipidaemia but with elevated C-reactive protein]. Revue medicale de Liege. 2008;63:749-53.

[19]	Ridker PM, Danielson E, Fonseca FA, Genest J, Gotto AM, Jr., Kastelein JJ, et al. Rosuvastatin to prevent vascular events in men and women with elevated C-reactive protein. *The New England journal of medicine.* 2008;359:2195-207.

[20]	Abbott AL. Medical (nonsurgical) intervention alone is now best for prevention of stroke associated with asymptomatic severe carotid stenosis: results of a systematic review and analysis. *Stroke; a journal of cerebral circulation.* 2009;40:e573-83.

[21]	Wennberg D, Lucas F, Birkmeyer J, Bredenberg C, Fisher E. Variation in carotid endarterectomy mortality in the Medicare population: Trial hospitals, Volume, and Patient Characteristics. *JAMA : the journal of the American Medical Association.* 1998;279:1278-81.

[22]	Conrad MF, Boulom V, Mukhopadhyay S, Garg A, Patel VI, Cambria RP. Progression of asymptomatic carotid stenosis despite optimal medical therapy. *Journal of vascular surgery.* 2013;58:128-35 e1.

[23]	Abbott A, Geroulakos G, Mikhailidis DP, Nicolaides AN, Sillesen H, Veith FJ. Regarding "Progression of asymptomatic carotid stenosis despite optimal medical therapy". *Journal of vascular surgery.* 2014;59:1752-3.

[24]	Kolos I, Loukianov M, Dupik N, Boytsov S, Deev A. Optimal medical treatment versus carotid endarterectomy: the rationale and design of the Aggressive Medical Treatment Evaluation for Asymptomatic Carotid

Artery Stenosis (AMTEC) study. International journal of stroke : *official journal of the International Stroke Society*. 2013.

[25] Reiff T, Bockler D, Bohm M, Bruckmann H, Debus ES, Eckstein HH, et al. Ongoing randomized controlled trials comparing interventional methods and optimal medical treatment in the treatment of asymptomatic carotid stenosis. *Stroke; a journal of cerebral circulation*. 2010;41:e605-6; author reply e7.

[26] Reiff T, Stingele R, Eckstein HH, Fraedrich G, Jansen O, Mudra H, et al. Stent-protected angioplasty in asymptomatic carotid artery stenosis vs. endarterectomy: SPACE2 - a three-arm randomised-controlled clinical trial. International journal of stroke : *official journal of the International Stroke Society*. 2009;4:294-9.

[27] Rothwell PM, Gibson R, Warlow CP. Interrelation between plaque surface morphology and degree of stenosis on carotid angiograms and the risk of ischemic stroke in patients with symptomatic carotid stenosis. On behalf of the European Carotid Surgery Trialists' Collaborative Group. *Stroke; a journal of cerebral circulation*. 2000;31:615-21.

[28] Mathiesen EB, Johnsen SH, Wilsgaard T, Bonaa KH, Lochen ML, Njolstad I. Carotid plaque area and intima-media thickness in prediction of first-ever ischemic stroke: a 10-year follow-up of 6584 men and women: the Tromso Study. *Stroke; a journal of cerebral circulation*. 2011;42:972-8.

[29] Takaya N, Yuan C, Chu B, Saam T, Underhill H, Cai J, et al. Association between carotid plaque characteristics and subsequent ischemic cerebrovascular events: a prospective assessment with MRI--initial results. *Stroke; a journal of cerebral circulation*. 2006;37:818-23.

[30] Singh N, Moody AR, Gladstone DJ, Leung G, Ravikumar R, Zhan J, et al. Moderate carotid artery stenosis: MR imaging-depicted intraplaque hemorrhage predicts risk of cerebrovascular ischemic events in asymptomatic men. *Radiology*. 2009;252:502-8.

[31] Altaf N, Daniels L, Morgan PS, Auer D, MacSweeney ST, Moody AR, et al. Detection of intraplaque hemorrhage by magnetic resonance imaging in symptomatic patients with mild to moderate carotid stenosis predicts recurrent neurological events. *Journal of vascular surgery*. 2008;47:337-42.

[32] Markus HS, King A, Shipley M, Topakian R, Cullinane M, Reihill S, et al. Asymptomatic embolisation for prediction of stroke in the Asymptomatic Carotid Emboli Study (ACES): a prospective observational study. *Lancet neurology*. 2010;9:663-71.

[33] Abbott AL, Chambers BR, Stork JL, Levi CR, Bladin CF, Donnan GA. Embolic signals and prediction of ipsilateral stroke or transient ischemic attack in asymptomatic carotid stenosis: a multicenter prospective cohort study. *Stroke; a journal of cerebral circulation.* 2005;36:1128-33.

[34] Molloy J, Markus HS. Asymptomatic embolization predicts stroke and TIA risk in patients with carotid artery stenosis. *Stroke; a journal of cerebral circulation.* 1999;30:1440-3.

[35] Orlandi G, Fanucchi S, Sartucci F, Murri L. Can microembolic signals identify unstable plaques affecting symptomatology in carotid stenosis? *Stroke; a journal of cerebral circulation.* 2002;33:1744-6; author reply -6.

[36] Siebler M, Nachtmann A, Sitzer M, Rose G, Kleinschmidt A, Rademacher J, et al. Cerebral microembolism and the risk of ischemia in asymptomatic high-grade internal carotid artery stenosis. *Stroke; a journal of cerebral circulation.* 1995;26:2184-6.

[37] Spence JD, Tamayo A, Lownie SP, Ng WP, Ferguson GG. Absence of microemboli on transcranial Doppler identifies low-risk patients with asymptomatic carotid stenosis. *Stroke; a journal of cerebral circulation.* 2005;36:2373-8.

[38] Markus HS, MacKinnon A. Asymptomatic embolization detected by Doppler ultrasound predicts stroke risk in symptomatic carotid artery stenosis. *Stroke; a journal of cerebral circulation.* 2005;36:971-5.

[39] King A, Markus HS. Doppler embolic signals in cerebrovascular disease and prediction of stroke risk: a systematic review and meta-analysis. *Stroke; a journal of cerebral circulation.* 2009;40:3711-7.

[40] Hirt LS. Progression rate and ipsilateral neurological events in asymptomatic carotid stenosis. *Stroke; a journal of cerebral circulation.* 2014;45:702-6.

Index

B

C

D